HOLISTIC HEALING IN TROPICAL DISEASES

by
Dr. Leo Rebello

Inputs from
Dr. Kashmira Rebello & Ms Dilnawaz Bana
on Anthroposophy & Eurythmy.
Dr. Firuzi Mehta & Dr. M.N. Sahukar
on Homeopathy.

NATURAL HEALTH CENTRE
Bombay, India

1

HOLISTIC HEALING IN TROPICAL DISEASES

© **Dr. Leo Rebello**

All Rights Reserved

First Edition, March 2006 / Second Edition, September 2013
ISBN-13: 978-1492243274 / ISBN-10: 1492243272

Proof reading: Dr. Kashmira Rebello
Typeset and designed by Actor Robin Rebello

MEDICAL BOOKS USUALLY CARRY A DISCLAIMER LIKE

"This book is meant purely for information purpose.
Readers are requested to consult experts before following the tips given here".

I CLAIM

That the knowledge contained in this book
is based on the collective wisdom of centuries.
It is to enlighten you and liberate you from the clutches of the medicine mafia.
The emphasis here is on "Your Health is in Your Hands".
Only in genuine emergencies you may go to the hospitals.
Otherwise, it is best that you remain far away from
doctors, drugs and death factories.
To accept this wise caution or not is entirely at your discretion.

I CLAIM

That this book has answers for everything on Health.
Holy books may not take you to Heaven,
but this book will certainly save your life from Hell.
Share these enlightened views with others.

Published by :
NATURAL HEALTH CENTRE
28/552 Samata Nagar, Kandivali (East), Bombay 400101, India.
Email: prof.leorebello@gmail.com Website: http://www.healthwisdom.org

Printed by CreateSpace

The front cover theme:

Dr. Sleep, Dr. Water, Dr. Exercise, Dr. Sunshine, Dr. Diet, Dr. Humour and Dr. Leo Rebello are the seven wonderful doctors of the world. If you follow their advice properly, you wlll live to be healthy hundred without ills, pills and hospital bills.

I am putting the second edition of this useful book in your hands, through CreateSpace's popular 'Print on Demand' and immediate dispatch scheme, which will make this book more accessible to the readers.

Several MDs, Holistic Healers, tourists, friends and students wrote or phoned from 2006 till date, that they immensely benefitted by the simple tips on diet, exercises, herbs, biochemic and homeopathic remedies given in this handybook. As such, they said, they could enjoy their holidays, business trips, long air and sea journeys.

Some said: This book is their regular companion in the handbag or by the bedside, for ready reference.

When this book was put on e-book platforms, it led to heavy piracy and we had to withdraw it. Hopefully, CreateSpace and Amazon should take care of this revenue loss to them as also to the authors.

I am a 'Doctor of Humanitarian Service' and believe that knowledge should be free, like all the God-given things are free. It is my experience though that the poor readily pay; but those who go into 'theft mode' do the mischief of downloading and violating someone's intellectual property rights.

For 'theft mentality' we have self-hypnosis through *Yoga* to help those with poor self-esteem, those who are generally bored, lonely and angry types, to delete their bad files. Incidentally, since Homeopathy also works on Body, Mind and Spirit Triad, we have very good remedies for overcoming stealing tendencies.

These Homeo Remedies Are: * *Calcarea Carb* (inclination to steal). * *Artemisia Vul* (habit of stealing in epilepsy). * *Stramonium* (habit of stealing in mania). * *Staphysagria* (general tendency to steal). * *Sulphur* (stealing habit in gamblers and tobacco smokers). * *Opium* (habit of thieving and telling lies).

Can the so-called scientific medicine claim, like Homeopathy, that they have medicines to change the stealing tendency? On the contrary, Allopathy creates criminals. By overdosing people with lethal drugs, aggression, depression, suicides, thefts, rapes, murders and other diseases multiply. Multi organ failures are on the rise, human organ thefts are on the rise.

This book repeats that *Health Care is Self Care*. Hence, break-free from the clutches of unscrupulous doctors as far as possible, so that you are not controlled and always be mobile, healthy and happy.

Namaste
Dr. Leo Rebello

3rd September 2013.

SELECT OPINIONS OF READERS

This book is my travel companion. Along with tickets, passport, credit card, it goes into my handbag, as I trust Dr. Leo Rebello, my Guru, completely. - **Anil Mehta, Yoga Teacher and Advocate, Bombay.**

Holistic Healing in Tropical Diseases is my trusted companion. I recommend it wholeheartedly to others. - **Jane MacRoss, Australia**

Dr. Leo Rebello, Ph.D., scholar from 1976-78 batch, has made outstanding contribution to Holistic Healing by writing several books and treating and training over a million people in 65 countries. We are proud of him. - **Dr. John Carson-Dunlop, Scotland.**

FOREWORD

The idea of writing a book on Tropical Diseases was planted in my mind by Dilnawaz Bana, who works at the Lucas Clinic for Cancer Research in Arlesheim, a beautiful town on the Swiss-German border. I have visited it three times, it being an ideal Cancer hospital. Dilnawaz's inputs on Remedial Eurythmy and Anthroposophic Medicine, jointly with my wife Kashmira, are appreciated.

As I decided to delve into the subject further, I found that tropical diseases were many. From 5 diseases which Dilnawaz had come up with initially, I increased the list to 15 to make this a traveler's complete companion and a guide to medical students, nurses and busy physicians.

The idea originally was to produce a booklet on Tropical Diseases. But it became a comprehensive compendium. Through this book a Total Picture of our Health unfolds. The idea is to make you responsible for your health rather than the doctors, and to warn you against drugs and the gargantuan hospitals.

Firuzi Dabu (a homeopath) and Minocher Sahukar (a retired dentist-homeopath-theosophist) provided much useful information and valuable insights enriching the value of this book.

Before we proceed further, always remember that blaming 'this germ' or 'that germ' and then attempting to kill it with potent medicines is unscientific. When we support that faulty line of modern medicine (a pseudo science), ignorance multiplies and consequently we become the promoters of wrong notions. To the best part of our ignorance that we arrange and classify we give the name 'knowledge'. My entire effort is to come out of this vicious circle and present full facts to the readers to empower them to challenge the orthodoxy and hegemony of modern medicine.

For example, how many doctors even know the symptoms of Yellow fever and claim to have treated it? Yet, people coming from 'yellow fever countries' are being quarantined (eventhough urban yellow fever has not been reported since 1942). There is also great scare about Anthrax, Ebola and Bird Flu. If one person dies of Bird Flu it becomes front page news. But millions dying due to alcohol or smoking is not even mentioned, because what will then happen to the advertisements from liquor barons and tobacco giants? The business of disease keeps everyone happy, except the patient. Even Bill Gates has now got onto the AIDS and Vaccines bandwagon, the most lucrative business.

I passed through Kuala Lumpur on way to Seoul in Korea during SARS paranoia and found check points in Malaysia, Singapore, Hong Kong and Bangkok. Disembarkation cards were accompanied with information sheets asking air travelers queer questions on sneezing, coughing etc. God-forbid if you were to strongly sneeze or cough, in front of the immigration counter while handing in the form, in which you said that you did not have cold, cough or fever, then the man in uniform could send you to SARS check point for quarantine and compulsory treatment. As a doctor, I had a good look at the SARS quarantine block, and am sorry to say that the men and women working there looked more like characters from a mental asylum, themselves frightened and frightening others. That is the kind of nonsense this modern medicine is. Create scare, sell medicines, weaken people, make them dependent and rake in profit.

Therefore, information has to be sifted into knowledge and knowledge into wisdom. Information can confuse, wisdom cannot. What the reader has to know is that drugs are not the answer to diseases. Drugs cannot cure diseases; drugs multiply them. A pure blood-stream is the answer.

HOLISTIC HEALING **is the ultimate wisdom.** If you were to follow the instructions given in this fine book, you will not have to depend on the devilish doctors and their witchcraft called modern medicine. *Ye Shall Know the Truth and the Truth Shall Make You Free.*

Dr. Leo Rebello

Bombay, February 21, 2006.

TROPICAL DISEASES
– An Introduction

Tropical diseases being widespread are difficult to prevent or control for various reasons - climate, poverty, primitive sanitation conditions and ignorance.

The most common diseases in the tropical regions are malaria, schistosomiasis, leprosy, filariasis, trypanosomiasis, and leishmaniasis. Both the infecting parasite and its mosquito carrier have become resistant to current drugs (chemotherapy and insecticides), and, it is estimated that about 500 million persons suffer from malaria in tropical areas.

Schistosomiasis has never been common in temperate climates, but it affects 200 million persons worldwide, and at least 20 percent are partly disabled by the disease.

Leprosy has always been more common in tropical climates, and about 20 million persons in the world have this illness. In endemic areas many severe cases of leprosy are now resistant to the drug first used against it.

Filariasis is a common tropical debilitating illness affecting an estimated 100 million persons. Trypanosomiasis, also known as sleeping sickness, results from infection with a protozoan. At least half a million people are affected. Leishmaniasis is also due to protozoan and can damage the internal organs. The World Health Organization estimates that worldwide some 12 million people are affected by leishmaniasis.

Tuberculosis is a considerable public health problem in much of the world and responsible for 2 million deaths annually, 75 percent of them in Asia. Other diseases include cholera, yellow fever, and amoebic dysentery.

Two forms of cancer, Burkitt's lymphoma and liver cancer are very common in Africa and Asia, respectively. Burkitt's lymphoma is usually due to malaria and liver cancer may be caused by infection with the hepatitis B virus.

As many as 25 million persons have become blind from preventable diseases in tropical countries. These diseases include xerophthalmia, due to lack of vitamin A in the diet; onchocerciasis, or river blindness, an infection of the skin by filarial larvae that may also affect the conjunctiva of the eye; and trachoma, a chronic conjunctival infection caused by the parasitic bacterium *Chlamydia trachomatis,* which is transmitted by flies or through close personal contact.

Finally, a number of severe fevers found predominantly in tropical regions include Lassa, Ebola, Marburg, Bunya, and Chikungunya fevers, some of which cause death by hemorrhage. The WHO estimates that there are some 50 million cases of dengue infection worldwide every year.

The severity of diseases in tropical areas is due to widespread poverty and poor sanitation as well as climatic influences. Poor sanitation is the root cause of cholera and schistosomiasis or for that matter all tropical diseases. Climate indirectly makes disease in tropical regions more severe by reducing agricultural production, which increases the risk of malnutrition. Hot weather and humid forests favour growth of the flies and mosquitoes that transmit malaria, yellow fever, trypanosomiasis and onchocerciasis.

Do not get frightened by the statistics of the diseases mentioned above. They are usually jacked up to push for more and more drugs. That is a well-laid out game plan of the Medicine Mafia. Also note that WHO is no more a World Health Organisation, but has degenerated into a WHOre of the Pharma cartel.

As Nobel Laureate Dr. Linus Pauling said, "Do not let either the medical authorities or the politicians mislead you. Find out what the facts are and make your own decisions about how to live a happy life and how to work for a better world".

I have traveled extensively in 65 countries and never been taken ill, as I am always cautious on what I eat, drink, about taking adequate rest, etc. I also carry essential homeopathy and biochemic remedies with me, along with common sense and conscience. It is best that you do the same and do not cross the limits.

TROPICAL COUNTRIES AND MEASURES TO PREVENT TROPICAL DISEASES

Tropical regions around the world are found in: Asia, Australia, Guam, Hawaii, New Caledonia, Nigeria, North America, Puerto Rico, South America, Tropic of Cancer and Tropic of Capricorn.

In the tropics, the intense sunlight heats the surface, which warms the air causing it to rise. This reduces the air pressure at the surface, forming a broad region of low pressure. As the warm, humid air rises, it often condenses into huge thunderstorms that provide the tropics with ample rainfall.

Temperature is an important aspect of climate and can be graded into five climatic zones: (1) Tropical, with annual and monthly averages above 20° C; (2) Subtropical, with 4 to 11 months above 20° C, and the balance between 10° and 20° C; (3) Temperate, with 4 to 12 months at 10° to 20° C; (4) Cold, with 1 to 4 months at 10° to 20° C, and the rest cooler; and (5) Polar, with 12 months below 10° C.

Asian countries share environmental problems due to rapid industrialization leading to serious air pollution. It also has some of the world's major health problems, compounded by widespread ignorance of basic sanitation concepts and, in some areas, by high population densities. Streams are often used for sewage disposal in the southern parts of Asia. These same streams are also used for drinking water and bathing. As such, they become a source of chronic infections.

The major diseases of Asia include cholera, typhoid fever, poliomyelitis, amoebic and bacillary dysentery, malaria and elephantiasis. Millions of people in Asia are infected with hookworms, which typically cause malnutrition, anemia and debilitation. Malnutrition itself causes diseases, including kwashiorkor, a protein deficiency disease that stunts the growth of children.

Construction of better drinking water facilities, together with improved systems of sewage disposal, rubbish collection and wastewater drainage, will create healthier settlements rather than pumping people with more and more drugs and weakening them further. It may also be noted that climate, different seasons, can have beneficial or adverse effects upon the human body. Hence, Ayurveda talks of seasonal foods and Chinese medicine talks of *Ying* and *Yang*, cold or hot food, balance.

Holistic Healing helps us in understanding the aetiology of illness and features common to the location or zone (the environmental factors). The primary causative factors are more useful than the cold microbiological facts and frightening parasitology. The natural immunity not based on the theory of 'antibodies in the blood' but the marvelous 'defense mechanism' or 'life force' is more important. Puddles of water, for example, will become mosquito breeding grounds. Therefore, instead of finding various ways of killing the mosquitoes, remove the stagnant water, the putrefying matter and mosquitoes will not breed. Likewise, simply killing the germs with more and more antibiotics or bactericidal agents may give temporary relief, but it does not help in removing the toxic wastes still festering in the system. A more resistant strain of bacteria is ever ready to thrive in such an environment.

So, if you are living in tropical countries or visiting them, then you are advised to take following precautions: * Do not go bare feet. * Always drink adequate clean water. * Instead of cokes, have coconut water. Try chilled coconut water and know the difference. * Have tropical fruits and lots of fresh fruit juices. * Wash your hands, face, feet before eating. * If you have come in contact with animals, in particular, dust your clothes, comb or brush your hair clean, wash your hands upto elbows, legs upto knees, wash face and only then eat. * Prefer clean and freshly cooked food to stale, refrigerated and recycled food. * Drink fresh buttermilk and eat curds (yogurt). That will protect your stomach and intestinal lining. * Use mosquito nets for sleeping in, where there is no airconditioning. * Use clothes that protect the body well or neem cream or eucalyptus oil on the skin. * Do not swim in polluted rivers, ponds or swimming pools which use chlorine; and above all do not drink the swimming pool water. * Avoid allopathic drugs, vaccinations and hospitals. * Trust homeopathic, biochemic and herbal medicines. * Do not panic.

HOLISTIC HEALING IN TROPICAL DISEASES

- Anthrax
- Cholera
- Dengue fever
- Dysentery (Bilharziasis or Schistosomiasis)
- Elephantiasis (Filariasis)
- Heat exhaustion and heat stroke
- Intestinal helminthiasis
- Jaundice (Hepatitis)
- Kala-azar
- Leprosy (Hansen's disease)
- Malaria
- Rabies (Hydrophobia)
- Tuberculosis
- Typhoid fever
- Yellow fever

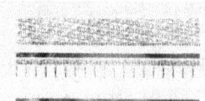

ANTHRAX

Anthrax is an acute, infectious disease caused by *Bacillus anthracis*, usually attacking cattle, sheep, horses, and goats. Those coming in contact with these animals and their hair, hides or waste can get infection through the skin, inhalation or per gastrointestinal tract. Anthrax can also be spread by eating undercooked meat of infected animals. Symptoms usually occur within 7 days.

Cutaneous: 95% anthrax infections occur when the bacterium enters a cut or abrasion on the skin. More commonly anthrax occurs as a pustule (boil) or itchy bump resembling an insect bite, exhibiting redness, vesiculation and induration with central ulceration, and development of black eschar. It may spread to lymph nodes and blood, and in some cases prove fatal. **Inhalational:** (rare) Symptoms like common cold develop leading to severe breathing problems and shock, if not attended to in time. **Intestinal** form of anthrax (also rare) is usually due to the consumption of contaminated meat or eating with unwashed hands after dealing with the animals or animal products. It is characterized by an acute inflammation of the intestinal tract. Nausea or vomiting, hyperpyrexia with headache are followed by abdominal pain, vomiting of blood, and severe diarrhea.

Allopathic doctors, after several inconclusive tests, will administer Penicillin or tetracycline in heavy doses, which will further sap the patient's strength and vitality and create additional diseases.

Nursing: For patients with inhalation anthrax, monitor vital signs and provide respiratory support. *Jala neti* (a yogic technique of nostril wash with lukewarm saline water) and induced sneezing will help. For cutaneous anthrax, keep lesions clean and cover the skin with sterile dressing of *Echinacea ointment.* Encourage oral fluid intake and offer lots of watery fruits, soups and small meals. Control hyperpyrexia through hydrotherapy, mud packs, compresses or herbal, homeopathic medicines as listed below. Application of Neem cream or turmeric paste on boils helps. Sunbathing in the morning sun and *pranayam* (deep breathing) or oxygen inhalation is useful.

Homeopathic remedies for Anthrax are: *Anthracinum* (a nosode or vaccine prepared from anthrax poison) should be the first remedy of choice, especially when there is epidemic spleen disease. Also when there is ulceration, intolerable burning, cyanosis and spasmodic breathing and with pustules on face and hands. Other remedies are: Arsenicum album, Carbo veg, Crotalus horridus, Hepar sulph, Secale cor, Tarentula cubensis, Veratrum album, Kreosotum, Lobelia inflata, Silicea, Stramonium.

Anthrax plagues farm animals and at times farm workers. Airborne Anthrax can be used by rogue nations as a biological weapon.

Anthrax spores attack the lungs.

Spores collect in the lymphnodes. Vaccines are not of much use.

Warrior cells or WBCs (body's defense) can kill spores only if the immunity is good.

Toxins further spread via the lymphatic system causing internal bleeding, damage to the organs. Antibiotics are of no use.

CHOLERA

Cholera is an acute, diarrheal illness caused by a short, curved, rod-shaped germ called, *Vibrio cholerae*. It is water borne disease more common at the end of summer and beginning of monsoon when flies multiply and water recedes and becomes heavy, putrid and contaminated. This is generally called the Cholera season.

The real cause of the disease, however, is the toxic and devitalized condition of the system brought about by incorrect food habits and faulty life style.

Approximately one in 20 infected persons has severe disease characterized by profuse watery diarrhea, vomiting and leg cramps. In these persons, rapid loss of body fluids leads to dehydration and shock. Death can occur within hours if proper treatment is not given.

Cholera spreads by drinking water mixed with sewage or eating contaminated food. The disease can spread rapidly in areas with inadequate treatment of sewage and drinking water. The cholera bacterium may also multiply in brackish rivers and coastal waters.

The disease is not likely to spread directly from one person to another; therefore, casual contact with an infected person is not a risk. When simple precautions are observed, contracting the disease is unlikely. Therefore, all travelers to areas where cholera has occurred should observe the following recommendations:

Drink only boiled water, and various hot teas, coffee or hot chocolates in milk. Avoid ice, ice creams, and chilled drinks. Eat only foods that have been thoroughly cooked and are still hot, or fruits that you have peeled yourself. Avoid undercooked or raw fish or shellfish. Make sure all vegetables are cooked; avoid salads. Lemon, onion, green chillies, vinegar and mint should be included in the daily diet during Cholera epidemic.

Cholera can be successfully treated by immediate replacement of the fluid and salts lost through diarrhea. Patients can be treated with oral rehydration solution (ORS), prepared by mixing a teaspoon of salt, 4 teaspoons of sugar (preferably honey), half a sour lime to one litre of warm water. This solution should be drunk in small sips at periodical interval. This solution is used throughout the world to treat diarrhea. Ready made ORS is also available with the chemists, but the said solution taken in large quantities will affect kidneys. Coconut water, lemon barley water, or fresh butter milk, fresh curds are also very good. Aloe vera juice may be taken with rehydrating drink. Severe cases may require intravenous fluid replacement. However, if the intravenous solution is old, spurious or substandard, then it may prove fatal. With prompt rehydration, cholera deaths can be 100% avoided.

Some home remedies are: *Nimbu Pani* (lemon water) sweetened with honey; leaves and flowers of peach, the leaves of drumstick, onion juice mixed with powder of black pepper and sweetened with honey applied in the mouth and then swallowed will give immediate results. The juice of bitter gourd (*karela*) may also be tried right at the onset.

Do not (repeat not) take antibiotics. Rather seek help of a good Homeopath or Naturopath if you are alone, confused, frightened and if do not have this book to refer to.

In the Cholera epidemic of 1830, Hahnemann ascribed its cause to "infinitely small, invisible living organisms". He published four pamphlets detailing the use of *camphor, cuprum* and *veratrum* for treatment of the epidemic. These give remarkable results. The other homeopathic remedies are: *Aconitum napellus,* to cut short cholera morbus. *Agaricus phalloides,* cramps in stomach, cold extremities, urine suppressed. *Ampelopsis quinquefolia,* violent vomiting and purging, with considerable tenesmus; then collapse, sweating, and faint pulse. *Apis mellifica,* cholera infantum with constant relapses, with threatening brain troubles, sunken abdomen, sunken fontanelle, which indicate dangerous condition. *Argentum nitricum,* sudden and severe attacks of cholera infantum; in children who are very fond of sugar, and who have eaten too much of it. *Arsenicum album,* cramps in the stomach, hands and lower half of forearm dark and livid, as in malignant cholera; constant vomiting and diarrhoea, with sharp nose, cold limbs, death-like condition. *Bryonia alba,* Cholera

Asiatica - vomiting and purging during cholera season, vomiting of food immediately after eating, skin is icy cold, shriveled, with pulselessness. *Carbo vegetabilis* may frequently be of service in the last stage of the disease, when the patient is in a state of collapse, or asphyxia, the pulse almost gone; the surface cold and bluish; the breath cold; or when the evacuations and cramps have ceased, and congestion to the chest takes place. *Plumbum metallicum,* in severe cases, particularly with spasms of abdominal muscles.

The biochemic remedies are: According to Schussler, the founder of biochemic remedies, in Cholera the specific remedy is *Natrum sulphuricum*. This remedy should be taken routinely as preventive, especially when you visit damp areas. Also: *Calcarea phosphoricum, Ferrum phosphoricum Kalium phosphoricum, Kalium sulphuricum, Magnesium phosphoricum* should be tried – all in 12X potency.

Breakfast

Lunch

Dinner

Breakfast

Lunch

Dinner

DENGUE FEVER

Dengue is a flu-like viral disease spread by the bite of infected mosquitoes. Dengue hemorrhagic fever is a severe, often fatal, complication of dengue. Prevention centers on avoiding mosquito bites and eliminating breeding sites.

Dengue is spread by the bite of an *Aedes* mosquito. The mosquito transmits the disease by biting an infected person and then biting someone else. This is the explanation given in the text books of Allopathy. Millions of *Aedes* mosquitoes may bite millions of people, why are only a few affected? Clearly this explanation does not convince. Also the allopathic treatment makes no sense. Sluggish blood is the cause and not *Aedes* mosquito *per se*.

Dengue viruses occur in most tropical areas of the world. Dengue is common in Africa, Asia, the Pacific, Australia, and the Americas. It is widespread in the Caribbean basin. Dengue is most common in cities but can be found in rural areas. It is rarely found in mountainous areas above 4,000 feet.

The mosquitoes that transmit dengue live among humans and breed in discarded tires, flower pots, old oil drums, and water storage containers close to human dwellings. Unlike the mosquitoes that cause malaria, dengue mosquitoes bite during the day.

Dengue fever usually starts suddenly with a high fever, rash, severe headache, pain behind the eyes, and muscle and joint pain. The severity of the joint pain has given dengue the name 'breakbone fever'. Nausea, vomiting, and loss of appetite are common. A rash usually appears 3 to 4 days after the start of the fever. The illness can last up to 10 days, but complete recovery can take as long as a month, if you use allopathic medicines. Adults are usually sicker than children.

Most dengue infections result in relatively mild illness, but some can progress to dengue hemorrhagic fever. Persons who were previously infected with dengue are thought to be at greater risk for developing dengue hemorrhagic fever if infected again.

With dengue hemorrhagic fever, the blood vessels start to leak and cause bleeding from the nose, mouth, and gums. Bruising can be a sign of bleeding inside the body. Without prompt treatment, the blood vessels can collapse, causing shock. Dengue hemorrhagic fever is fatal in about 5 percent of cases.

Dengue is diagnosed by a blood test. There is no specific treatment for dengue in modern medicine. Persons with dengue fever should rest and drink plenty of fluids. They should be kept away from mosquitoes for the protection of others. Dengue hemorrhagic fever is treated by replacing lost fluids. Some patients need transfusions to control bleeding.

Avoid mosquito bites when traveling in tropical areas: by using mosquito repellents on skin and clothing, by wearing long-sleeved shirts and long pants tucked into socks. When indoors, stay in air-conditioned or screened areas. Use bednets if sleeping areas are not screened or air-conditioned.

Eliminate mosquito breeding sites around homes. Discard items that can collect rain or run-off water, especially old tires. Regularly change the water in outdoor bird baths and pet and animal water containers.

Homeopathic Eupatorium perfoliatum could be considered as a specific for dengue. According to Dr. R.L.Gupta, *Aconite-30* alternated by *Ipecac-30* works very well in dengue fever with vomiting, nausea and anxiety. *Arsenicum album* is effective in dengue fever with diarrhoea and thirst; great debility, exhaustion and restlessness, worse at night; sudden sinking of strength, fear of death; intense headaches, worse from light and noise, better by wrapping up warm; small offensive dark stools with great prostration; dark, offensive haemorrhage from bowels during dengue haemorrhagic fever. Then there is *Belladonna* which works in high fever, red hot face, red eyes, hot head, puffy eyes, bleeding from inner parts, uncontrollable vomiting. *Colocynthis,* soreness in bones; aching of bones, with soreness of the flesh; bruised feeling in every bone preventing lying in bed and causing despair, moaning and crying out. These "bone pains" are the characteristics of this ancient domestic remedy. *Nux vomica, i*rritable, hypersensitive and over-impressionable; stools often mixed with mucous and blood; blue mottled spots on skin during fever; aching in limbs and back with fever.

According to Dr. William Boericke's Repertory and Materia Medica, remedies commonly used for dengue are: Aconite; Arsenic album; Belladonna; Bryonia; Cantharis; China; Eupatorium; Gelsemium; Ipecac; Nux vomica; Rhus tox and Rhus venenata.

Biochemic Remedies: Dr. R.L.Gupta recommends a combination of the four biochemic remedies, namely, *Ferrum phosphoricum, Kalium muriaticum, Natrum muriaticum, Natrum sulphuricum* along with the indicated homeopathic remedy in cases of dengue.

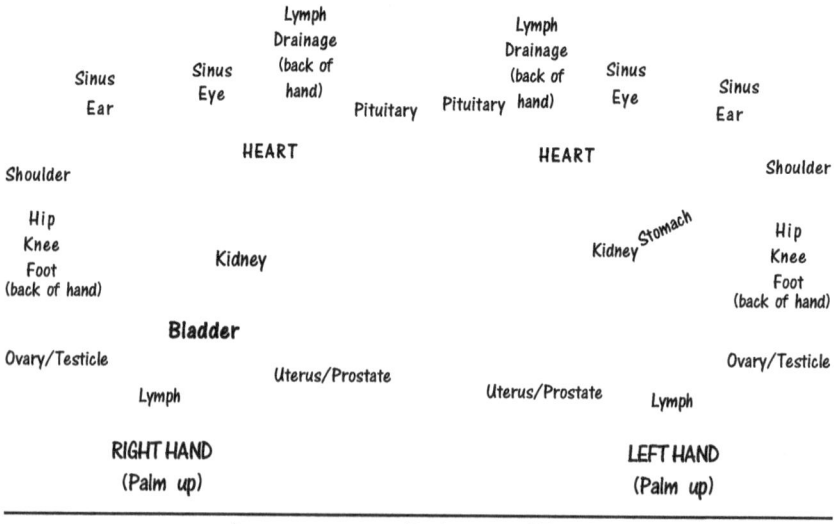

Accupressure Points on Hands

DYSENTERY

Dysentery is a serious condition affecting the large intestine. It is accompanied by inflammation and ulceration of the bowel, a colicky pain in abdomen and passing of liquid or semi-formed stools with mucus and blood. The pathological condition is caused by two organisms, protozoa and bacilli. The one caused by protozoa is known as *Amoebic dysentery* and the other is called *Bacillary dysentery.* Dysentery occurs all over the world, except in very cold regions. People living in squalid surroundings will be more prone to it and children in particular, eventhough it can affect anyone.

Amoebiasis is caused by *E. histolytica* commonly spread by water contaminated by faeces or from food served by dirty hands. Even vegetables, if not washed or cooked properly, may transmit the disease. Initially, the patients have lower abdominal pain and diarrhoea and later develop dysentery (with blood and mucus in stool). Fulminant infection with high-grade fever, severe abdominal pain and profuse diarrhoea occurs in children and in patients receiving steroids. Severe gastric distention of the bowel can occur. Amoebomas (inflammatory mass lesion developing in chronic amoebiasis) can present like a malignancy. If it affects the liver, it causes pus formation.

Another type of Dysentery is known as Bilharziasis or Schistosomiasis. This is the parasitic (Fluke) dysentery. Allopathy has drug Praziquantel, which is costly and has side effects like chills, contractures, muscles pains, great prostration and faintness, sweating, convulsive twitching, cough and yawning consecutively. Treatment is worse than the disease. 200 million people are infected worldwide, according to statistics available.

Fasting is the best remedy in severe cases of dysentery. Generally fast of two days should provide rest for the gastro-intestinal tract. During fasting, the patient should take orange juice, carrot juice, pomegranate juice, coconut water, buttermilk, barley water, and warm water to establish helpful micro-organisms in the intestines. Small doses of castor oil in the form of emulsion will act as a mild aperient and facilitate expulsion of offensive matter. After the acute symptoms are over the patient may be allowed *Kanji* (see Annexures section), rice and curd, fresh ripe fruits, especially bael, banana and pomegranate. Garlic, which is a natural antibiotic, will aid digestion and expel parasites. It should be eaten with bananas.

Turmeric is another easily available natural remedy. It is a useful intestinal antiseptic and gastric tonic. Mix turmeric powder with honey and apply on the tongue. It can also be taken mixed with water or buttermilk. Lemon juice mixed in boiled water and taken periodically also helps considerably. Honey taken with cinnamon powder will give relief in stomach ache and intestinal ulcers, if any.

Ginger compress, mud compress or wet towel on the abdomen will relieve cramps. Drink Ginseng tea if available and eat one salted plum a day for about a month to strengthen the digestive tract. *Pawan Muktasan, Paschimtanasan, Ardha Matsyendrasan* and *Nauli Kriya* (these specific abdomen pressing yoga postures) will help.

Pawan Muktasan   Paschimtanasan   Ardha Matsyendrasan

Meats of all kinds, silver fish and shell fish (which are carrier of amoebas) should be avoided for at least six months. Likewise, tea, coffee, alcohol, cokes should be desisted to avoid relapse.

The important homeopathic remedies are: Aconitum napellus, Aloes, Alstonia, Arsenicum album, Baptisia tinctoria, Belladonna, Carbo vegetabilis, Cinchona officinalis, Colocynthis, Emetin, Erigeron, Mercurius corrosivus, Nux vomica, Sulphur. *Biochemic Remedy that works wonders in Dysentery is Kali phos 6X.*

ELEPHANTIASIS

Elephantiasis or Filariasis is prevalent in tropical Africa, Indonesia, the South Pacific, coastal Asia, southern Arabia, southern Mexico and Gautemala. It is a chronic infectious condition caused by roaming bare feet in the Red soil, aggravated by mosquitoes and leading to massive swelling of legs, arms and the scrotum, with thickening and darkening of the overlying skin. As it resembles the skin of an elephant it is called elephantiasis or pachydermatosis. Largely it is due to chronic lympathic obstruction occurring as a feature of filariasis, caused by microscopic worms, such as, *Wuchereria bancrofti, Brugia malayi,* and *B. timori.* It may also be congenital (Milroy's disease).

The cycle of filariasis: **(a)** larvae enter the body through the bite of blood-sucking insect; **(b)** larvae spread throughout the body via the bloodstream and lymphatic vessels; **(c)** in the lymphatics, larvae develop into adult worms, which produce more larvae; **(d)** the new larvae enter the blood and are ingested by a blood-sucking insect.

Swollen lymphnodes and recurring attacks of fever are early acute symptoms. Inflammation of lymph vessels results in localized oedema (an accumulation of liquid in the tissues, causing swelling). Following repeated infections, the affected area, commonly the limb or the scrotum, becomes enormously enlarged and the skin becomes thick, coarse and fissured.

Fever, chills and a general feeling of ill health (malaise) may be present. The penis may be retracted under skin, which has become thickened, non-elastic, hot and painful.

The spermatic cords may become thickened. The external parts of the female genitalia (vulva) may also be affected. Enlargement of the lymph nodes of the legs and death of surrounding tissues leading to gangrene are other complications.

The diagnosis of Filariasis is confirmed by microscopic examination of the blood for the presence of microfilarae. A three week course of the *anthelminthic drug, diethylcarbamazine,* works during acute exacerbation, but may cause a reaction marked by fever, sickness and muscle and joint pains.

Colonic irrigation, followed by three days fasting, ingestion of neem leaves, drum stick leaves, and raw fruit diet for about three months, fresh buttermilk with coriander (no salt), lymphatic drainage massage, application of turmeric on the affected parts, externally, and homeopathic and biochemic medicines, internally, will bring excellent results.

Homeopathic and biochemic remedies indicated are:

Arsenicum album: Elephantiasis, with burning pains and enormous swelling of the limb, or with ulcerations; itching, burnings, swellings. *Bixa orellana:* a South American herb that's related to the *Chaulmoogra* plant, recommended for leprosy, eczema and elephantiasis. *Carduus marianus:* Varicose veins, ulcers and oedema of the feet. *Hippozaeninum (Glanderinum, Nosode of Glanders)* - For inflammation of veins and lymphatics esp., if pus is formed, all the attacked parts swell. *Hydrastis canadensis:* Extensive oedema of ankle and foot, elephantiasis with deep spreading ulcers. *Iodium:* Acts prominently on nodosities, enlarged glands, bleeding ulcers, hectic fever. *Ledum palustre:* Ailments from bites and stings, elephantiasis of lower limbs. *Myristica sebifera:* This remedy has a decided action in the relief of elephantiasis arabum. *Rajania subsamarata* - Ulcerous vulvar elephantiasis. *Silicea:* Elephantiasis in general and of scrotum. Biochemic remedy for elephantiasis is *Calcarea fluoricum* 12X four hourly.

HEAT EXHAUSTION AND HEAT STROKE

Heat exhaustion is an acute heat injury with hyperthermia caused by dehydration. It occurs when the body no longer can dissipate heat adequately because of extreme environmental conditions or increased endogenous heat production. It may progress to heatstroke when the body's thermoregulatory mechanisms become overwhelmed and fail. It may lead to end-organ damage with universal involvement of the CNS.

Heatstroke traditionally is divided into exertional and classic types. Exertional heatstroke typically occurs in younger athletic patients who exercise vigorously in the heat. Classic heatstroke more commonly occurs in older patients or in patients with underlying illnesses who are exposed to extreme environmental conditions.

When heat is generated or gained by the body faster than it can be dissipated, heat illness occurs. The body's basal metabolic rate is 50-60 kcal/h/m^2. The body's dominant forms of heat loss in a hot environment are radiation (65%) and evaporation (30%). The remaining is through conduction and convection.

Heat exhaustion signs: Fatigue and weakness, nausea and vomiting, headache and myalgias, dizziness, muscle cramps and irritability. The critical feature of heatstroke is CNS dysfunction, which has a sudden onset in 80% of cases. Symptoms include profuse sweating, bizarre behavior, hallucinations, altered mental state, confusion, disorientation, trembling and coma. The patient's temperature is usually higher than 106°F (41°C) – at that temperature brain cells are damaged if the temperature is not brought down immediately.

Exercise in a hot environment, lack of air conditioning or proper ventilation, inappropriate clothing (eg, occlusive, heavy, vapor-impermeable), lack of acclimatization, decreased fluid intake, hot environments (eg, inside of tents or autos in the sun, hot tubs, saunas) can increase heat. Drugs and toxins like beta-blockers, anticholinergics, diuretics, ethanol, antihistamines, cyclic antidepressants, sympathomimetics (eg, cocaine, amphetamines), phenothiazines, lithium and salicylates will further escalate the problem, as also salt or water depletion and obesity.

Heatstroke affects almost every organ in the body except the pancreas. If not treated immediately, it may also affect the brain, heart and blood, lungs, liver and kidneys. However, with rapid cooling, adequate rehydration, and immediate treatment of complications, the recovery and survival rate in heatstroke is almost 100%.

In any emergency, it is the First Aid or prehospital care which is more important. The mainstay of therapy involves prompt cooling. Remove the patient from the hot environment and transfer to a shady place, a cool vehicle, or a cool building. Fan the patient, or pour water on the head, or apply ice packs to the patient's neck, axillae, and groin. Alternatively, cover the patient with a wet sheet. Give cold fruit juices, cold coconut water, cold lemon barley, cold *Nimbu Pani* (sour lime water with sugar or honey) or cold *Jal Jeera* (cumin seeds powder added to water, with a little salt and sugar) to drink. Cold water colonic irrigation is advised. No stimulants (alcohol, etc.) should be given. Body fluid replacement in extreme dehydration, with saline intravenous drip may be permissible.

Homeopathic medicines for heat exhaustion/stroke are:
Aconite napellus: Complaints from very hot weather, rapid and sudden onset of symptoms. *Agaricus muscarius:* Vertigo and head ache from exposure to sun. *Anacardium orientale:* Temporary loss of memory after sunstroke. *Belladonna:* Weakness and unconsciousness following sunstroke. *Carbo vegetabilis:* Faintness from sunstroke, head pain, nausea and diarrhoea from heat of sun. *Glonoinum:* Weakness from sunstroke, clenched jaw and eyes staring, unconsciousness, loss of memory, vertigo, congestion of the head, intermittent headaches and fever. *Nux vomica:* Confusion of mind in the sun, head pain from sun exposure. *Selenium:* Headpain from sun exposure, skin sensitive to the sun; sunburn and general weakness from heat of the sun.

Biochemic remedies are: *Natrum muriaticum* and *Kalium phosphoricum* in 6X at half hourly interval.

Once a patient is admitted in a hospital, instead of treating the patient on emergency basis, they will advise several costly and time-wasting Lab Studies like CBC, PT, aPTT, Electrolytes, BUN, and creatinine, blood glucose, creatine kinase, arterial blood gases, urinalysis, chest x-ray, CT scan of the head. And various consultants will prescribe drugs according to their limited understanding.

For God's sake avoid these drugs: *Anticholinergics* (given to decrease sweating), *alpha-adrenergic agonists* (given to increase peripheral resistance without increasing cardiac output), and *antipyretics* (which will not help decrease body temperature as it is not due to fever). *Salicylates* can worsen coagulopathies, and *acetaminophen* in large doses can worsen hepatic damage. *Neuroleptics* may lead to bone marrow suppression; narrow-angle glaucoma; severe liver or cardiac damage. Other *CNS depressants, anticholinergics, anticonvulsants,* or *antihypertensives* may cause significant hypotension and Parkinsonism. *Benzodiazepines,* which are unsafe in pregnancy, may lead to respiratory depression and toxicity. *Diuretics,* which are used to promote diuresis and prevent or treat acute renal failure, may lead to anuria; severe pulmonary congestion; severe dehydration; active intracranial bleeding; progressive renal damage; progressive heart failure. As I have said time and again, in hospitals you get more diseases. Not for nothing Ayurveda calls Doctors, Yama's younger brothers. (*Yama* is Hindu death God).

INTESTINAL HELMINTHIASIS

There are over 3200 varieties of intestinal parasites.
Testing is available for about one percent of the known varieties
with about twenty-percent accuracy.

Helminthiasis (intestinal parasites/worms) which infest human beings are found in all countries of the world. However, they are more common in tropical and subtropical areas and are widely prevalent during the rainy season. There are four types of intestinal worms, namely, hook worm, tape worm, thread worm and round worm.

TAPEWORM

female

male

SEATWORM

ROUNDWORM

female

male

HOOKWORM

There can be hundreds of varieties / of parasites / worms living in human bodies. Not all of them are harmful. Parasitic worms can invade our bodies through food and water intake, through a transmitting agent (like a mosquito), sexual conduct or through the nose and skin. Once established, they will eat the same foods you eat or they will eat you.

The eggs of these parasites are introduced into the human system through the medium of contaminated food or water. All meats, old meats (beef and pig, in particular) are the breeding ground for worms. Hookworms enter the human body through bare foot walking on infected earth. Tapeworms are transmitted to the body through contaminated, stale, under cooked flesh foods or foods contaminated by dogs. You are at a higher risk in contracting worms when pets are allowed indoors. Dogs and cats are host to many parasites that humans can contract. Animals can spread 240 diseases to humans because of parasites.

People, especially small children, with intestinal parasites (*verminous intoxification*) will have bloated abdomen due to digestive disorders; they will be under-nourished and weak as they can destroy cells faster than they are regenerated. People with worm infestation may also suffer from anemia, asthma, low immune system, fatigue, nervousness, foul breath, dark circles under the eyes, and restlessness at night with bad dreams, headaches, rash, fever etc. Human intestinal parasites can be present in any disease, in any person, at any age.

The real cause of intestinal worms, however, is faulty living. These parasites and the eggs of these worms can breed in intestines only if they find there a suitable medium for their propagation. The medium is an intestinal tract clogged with morbid matter.

Allopathy treats with *Perazine (Antepar or Pripsen)* or *Mebendazole (Vermox)*. It claims that a single oral dose of *Niclosamide (Yomesan)* will eradicate the worm infestation.

In Naturopathy we prescribe Garlic, Carrots and Pumpkin seeds to clear the worms. Castor oil will flush them out in one go, followed by a day's fast on carrot juice and chewing of garlic pods. Neem juice enema too works wonders. Pumpkin seeds and onions mixed with soy milk is another remedy for worms. Fasting on raw pineapples for three days helps expel tapeworms. Use more cloves with every meal. Adding cloves to foods will help kill the eggs from parasites in the intestinal tract. Another remedy for prevention is mixing one or two teaspoons of apple cider vinegar in a glass of water. Alternatively, you can take one tablespoon daily of 1 part apple cider vinegar, 2 parts apple juice, 1 part apple brandy.

Homeopathic Treatment: E.A.Farrington in *Comparative Materia Medica* records, "Recourse must be taken to the deep-acting, constitutional, anti-psoric remedies to eradicate the verminous diathesis. They must be prescribed on general constitutional basis, without ever thinking of prescribing for the worms. They will so correct the constitution that order will be established in the interior economy of the body and the worms will no longer hatch out".

The ringworm parasites are of the mold or vegetable order and one of the consumption nosodes, notably *Bacillinum,* is the basic remedy. Burnett noticed that when prescribing a course of *Scirrhinum* and other cancer nosodes for patients this was often followed by the expulsion of worms.

This observation indicates that the liability to intestinal parasites may be one symptom of the cancerous diathesis, and it also suggests that *Scirrhinum 30,* once or twice a week should be included among the constitutional remedies for helminthiasis.

H.N.Guernsey, in *Diseases of Children,* explains: "Worms constitute one of the most common disorders of children. And people imagine that, if the worms are expelled their children will be cured. But this is a great mistake; for children are not ill so much because they have worms, as they have worms because they are ill". Then he rightly adds: "Consequently the violent medicines, drugs, and even mechanical means used to destroy and expel the worms, either entirely fail of their object or, in effecting it, inflict still greater injury upon the health. The indications afforded by the symptoms enable the Homeopathic physician to prescribe the remedy for the entire disordered condition which leads to the development of the worms themselves. Besides, in many cases of supposed 'worms', they in reality do not produce the sufferings". Guernsey further elaborates: "There are two kinds of worms to which children are liable; the lumbricoides, or long round worms, and the ascarides, or pin-worms. The latter principally infest the rectum. Besides these there are occasionally cases of tapeworm, tænia; but these seldom occur in small children".

Main homeopathic medicines in worms are:

Arsenicum album: Ascarides lumbricoides, oxyuris vermicularis, trichinae; vomiting of worms. *Belladonna:* Convulsions from worms, drowsiness, grating of teeth, involuntary micturition and defaecation; squinting. *Calcarea carbonica:* it is a valuable constitutional remedy to eradicate the disposition to worms. *Carboneum sulphuratum:* for pinworms, roundworms, tapeworms. *Chamomilla:* Fever, diarrhea, sleeplessness or convulsions from roundworms. *Cicuta virosa:* Convulsions in children from worms. The patient is suddenly rigid, with fixed staring eyes, bluish face, frothing at the mouth and unconscious. There are shocks and jerks through the body, frequent hiccough and crying, pain in the neck, dilated pupils, spasmodic drawing of the head backwards, tremor of hands, constriction of oesophagus; weakness with worms. *Cina maritima:* Most powerful for the elimination of roundworms. The sickly appearance of the face, the blue rings about the eyes and the grinding of the teeth, rubbing of the nose, associated with canine hunger and itching of anus is the perfect picture of Cina. *Cucurbita pepo:* This is a specific and special poison to the taenia (tape worm). *Cuprum oxydatum nigrum:* Zopfy, in his sixty years' practice, asserts that this remedy will remove all kinds of worms, cure trichinosis, and even tapeworm. He gives it in small doses, about the 1x, in alternation with *Nux vomica* four or five times a day for four to six weeks, which always suffices to cure tapeworm without causing the patient any inconvenience whatever. *Lycopodium clavatum:* Ascarides with much rumbling in the bowels, or red sand in the urine. *Spigelia anthelminthica:* Strabismus, stammering (repeats first syllable three or four times) due to helminthiasis and other abdominal ailments. *Thymolum:* Specific for hookworm disease.

Natrium phosphoricum is the principal Biochemic remedy for all kinds of worms. Pain in the bowels, restless sleep, picking at nose, itching of rectum and grinding of teeth; with acidity. *The other Biochemic remedies are: Calcarea fluorica:* long, round, or thread-worms with characteristic symptoms of acidity, occasional squinting; pain in the bowels, restless sleep. Itching of the anus, face white about the mouth or nose. Grinding of the teeth in children. This remedy probably acts by destroying the excess of lactic acid which seems to be necessary for the life of these worms. *Ferrum phosphoricum:* thread worms, predisposition to passing undigested food.

R.L.Gupta in *Directory of Diseases and Cures in Homeopathy* prescribes the following medicines for worms.

For roundworms: Abrotanum, Aesculus hippocastanum, Antimonium crudum, Chelone, Cina, Granatum, Helminthochortos, Ignatia, Lycopodium, Mercurius dulcis, Passiflora incarnata, Sabadilla, Santoninum, Spigelia, Stannum, Teucrium marum, Urtica urens. *For threadworms:* Arsenic album, Baptisia, Chelone,

Cina, Ignatia, Lycopodium, Mercurius dulcis, Mercurius sulphuricus, Natrum phosphoricum, Ratanhia, Santoninum, Sinapis nigra, Teucrium marum, Valeriana. *For tapeworms:* Cucurbita, Filix mas, Granatum, Kuosso, Sabadilla, Sabin, Santoninum, Stannum, Valeriana. *For hookworms:* Abrotanum, Aesculus, Arsenic album, Baptisia, Calcarea carbonica, Chelone, Cina, Ferrum mur, Filix mas, Granatum, Ignatia, Kousso, Lycopodium, Naphthaline, Natrum phosphoricum, Passiflora incarnata, Pulsatilla, Ratanhia, Sabadilla, Santoninum, Spigelia, Stannum, Sumbul, Teucrium marum.

Hygienic Treatment: Keep your fingernails short, wash your rectum in the morning, bathe and change your underwear. Wash your hands thoroughly before eating. Uncooked or undercooked fish or meat should be avoided to guard against worm-infestation. Sweets, sugar, pastry, unwashed fruits and vegetables, not grown organically, should be avoided. Children suffering from thread-worms should be prevented from putting their fingers into their mouth, as they are very apt to scratch the irritated parts in sleep. This caution may be necessary for older persons as well.

Healthy immune system is the best defense against parasites and disease. Here are some of the additional things you can do to reduce the risk of parasitic infestations.

Washing in ozonated water, hydrogen peroxide (1 teaspoon per gallon of water), or bleach (add 1/2 teaspoon to each gallon and soak for 10 minutes) will kill parasites. Rinse well to remove bleach residue. Don't use chlorine water to clean fruits, as chlorine is carcinogenic.

Thoroughly cook meats and fish. Do not eat raw or uncooked meats or fish. Check for worms, especially on fish. Spray with hydrogen peroxide or wash in ozonated water before cooking. Keep all work surfaces clean.

Drink pure water. Water that is properly purified with ozone is free of parasites.

Practice good personal hygiene. Wash your hands before eating and after going to the bathroom, changing diapers, or handling pets. Keep your fingernails short and clean. Parasites (eggs) can live for two months under the fingernails.

Do not walk barefoot on warm, moist soil or while working in the garden. Parasites are abundant in soil and can penetrate through skin cells. Fertilizers are added to garden soil and it is the pets' favorite place to go. Use gloves and shoes for protection.

Swimming in rivers, lakes, ponds, or public swimming pools should be avoided. Avoid swallowing or drinking the water while swimming anywhere. Avoid swimming if cuts or open sores are present.

Overuse of antibiotics. Reducing the numbers of friendly bacteria in the colon allows for the proliferation of parasites.

Most effective treatment or cleansing product for the elimination of parasites in the large intestine is to cleanse the colon with ozonated water and hydrogen peroxide by colonic irrigation. This method is extremely beneficial to expel all types of bad bacteria, food pathogens, parasites and viruses.

As the colon becomes cleaner, the ozone and oxygen will reach other organs where parasites may be a problem. Why does ozone work so well? Healthy cells and friendly bacteria are aerobic, which means they need oxygen to survive. Unhealthy cells, parasites, pathogens and viruses are anaerobic, they can survive in a non oxygenated environment. Change their living environment and you win the war.

JAUNDICE

Jaundice (also called the yellow disease or hepatitis) is nothing but malfunctioning or inflammation of the liver due to many reasons – typhoid, malaria, yellow fever, tuberculosis, alcohol consumption and accumulations of various toxins due to poor digestion. Jaundice assumes epidemic proportions in over-crowded places, dirty surroundings leading to contamination of water and food.

In jaundice the patient's skin and white of the eyes (sclera) turn yellow. Even the urine turns yellow and smells foul. This is due to the presence of bilirubin in the blood stream. Bilirubin is produced in the spleen when old or damaged red blood cells (RBCs) are destroyed. Normally, the liver passes the pigment into the intestine and out through faeces. There are various reasons why bilirubin may accumulate in the blood, causing jaundice. It could be due to liver cancer, cirrhosis, or hepatitis; or gall stones in the bile duct, which block the outflow of bile from the liver, preventing the excretion of bilirubin. If yellowing is due to cancer of liver or gallstones, the treatment should be accordingly. Gall bladder stones can be expelled (non surgically) with Olive Oil and Lemon treatment within 24 to 48 hours.

Jaundice can be recognised by the following symptoms: low fever initially, sensitivity to smells, nausea/vomiting, lack of appetite, back pain, general malaise, yellowing of skin, eyes, nails, urine, clay coloured stools, giddiness and headache. The patient may also feel a dull pain in the liver region.

Inspite of the jaundice signs being so obvious, doctors of modern medicine will further put the patients to heavy expenses by asking them to undertake urine tests, blood tests, x-rays or scan of the gall bladder or liver. They won't reveal that they get 'cuts' from all these tests, but will assure you that these tests are necessary to determine the cause of the disease. After that what? Steroids? Glucose saline? Vitamins?

The most common type of jaundice is hepatitis-A. Patients usually recover within three weeks without any specific treatment. Hepatitis-B is considered fatal. The cause is usually a vaccine laced with mercury. So, beware of Hepatitis-B vaccine if you wish to live long. First the said vaccine was available for Rs.600, now it is Rs.50 (subsidised). It is a big racket like polio dose.

Sometimes, healthy babies too suffer from jaundice during the first week of life (congenital). This condition is not serious and quickly passes. It is a normal result of the destruction of excess RBCs not needed once the baby can breathe. Don't allow your tiny tots to be jabbed for blood. Because, more children get jaundice in hospitals due to unsterilised needles, and surroundings, including unhygienic delivery room.

When bile does not reach the duodenum due to blockage or liver cell changes, spleen enlarges and this can be fatal if not treated properly. There is another kind of jaundice called toxic jaundice resulting from toxic substances, such as, phosphorus, arsphenamine, carbon tetrachloride.

Allopathy has absolutely no answer to Jaundice whether A or B or obstructive jaundice or cirrhosis of liver. They have labeled Jaundice as a highly infectious and notifiable disease. That means you have to shift the patient (technically) to an Infectious Diseases Hospital, where the patient may get more diseases due to cross infection.

Jaundice has become a big business (literally) for the practitioners of modern medicine who have nothing much to offer in jaundice and yet will make big *hoo-haa* out of it by their scientific jargon and battery of tests. Instead of educating the masses, they will frighten them so that the patients become dependent on them. This is their usual *modus operandi*. Therefore, do NOT listen to them and treat the patient at home by taking adequate precaution.

Nature Cure advises treating liver imbalance by avoiding fats, alcohol and drugs. Drink 2 or 3 glasses daily of fresh vegetable juices, particularly celery or carrot. Put mudpack or warm castor oil compress on the liver region, give warm water enema to evacuate large intestine of faecal material.

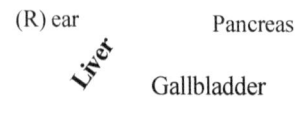

FOOT REFLEX POINTS

Pituitary

Stiff neck

(R) eye

(R) ear

Liver

Pancreas

Gallbladder

Absolutely no meats during jaundice attack. Massage can also be given to the reflex areas relating to the liver and gall bladder and also to areas relating to the solar plexus and the adrenal and pituitary glands.

Banana, more particularly yellow banana is a panacea in jaundice. Slice it, add a pinch of turmeric powder and give at least once a day. Similarly, intake of papaya, green grams, sugar cane to chew, buttermilk with coriander, coconut water, and lots of water to drink will bring excellent results within 3 to 5 days, as toxins will be flushed out per urine and faeces.

Home Remedies: (a) A teaspoon of tamarind pulp, jaggery and cumin taken thrice daily will cure jaundice, nausea, vomiting, and giddiness. **(b)** Soak two tablespoons of dry fenugreek (*methi*) seeds in a glassful of water for about four hours. Then boil the water till it is reduced to ¼ the quantity. Strain this decoction through muslin cloth and add a tablespoon of pure honey to it. Give this tonic medicine for seven consecutive nights. **(c)** Extract juice of green leaves of radish and let the patient drink at least one glass midmorning daily for about ten days to flush out all toxins from the body.

Yoga for Jaundice: Do *yogic kriyas* like nasal irrigation, eyewash, mouthwash and stomach wash. Deep breathing and *surya namaskar,* liver and gallbladder compressing asanas like *paschimtanasan, halasan, ardha matsyendrasan, dhanurasan, makarasan* are very beneficial in Jaundice.

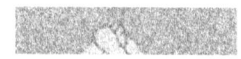

Halasan   Makarasan   Dhanurasan

In Homeopathy, we have many medicines for Jaundice

(a) *Aconite 30* / 4 pills thrice a day (tds): Jaundice during pregnancy.

(b) *Chamomilla 30* / 4 hourly. Infantile Jaundice: newborn baby cries a lot.

(c) *Ipecac 30* / 4 hourly: In the beginning when there is nausea and vomiting.

(d) *China 30* / tds: Liver swollen and sensitive.

(e) *Nux vomica 30:* jaundice due to constipation, alcoholism, and gastric complaints. It is also 'the remedy' for Hepatitis B and should be given for atleast 15 days to remove the disease taint.

(f) *TNT 200* / 4 pills once a week for about a month, for Haemolytic jaundice.

(g) Intercurrent remedy: *Sulphur 30* / 4 pills once a week, for about a month.

Other homeopathic remedies for jaundice are: Carduus marianus, Chelidonium, Lachesis, Arsenic album, Podophyllum, Iodium, Leptandra, Phosphorus (all in 30 or 200 potencies) **and the biochemic remedies are:** *Ferrum phosphoricum, Kali muriaticum and Natrum sulphuricum,* in 6x potencies.

In Ayurveda a well-known medicine for Liver disorders and Jaundice is: Liv 52 (tablets, syrup and drops), which even Allopaths prescribe. But it is no longer the No.1, as it used to be 10 years ago. Other herbal and ayurvedic medicines, equally or more effective, are catching up with Liv 52.

If it is Jaundice, the *mantra* is do not trust the newspapers, health officials and allopathic doctors, who create panic. Boil the water; eat fresh food and fruits which are not exposed. No refrigerated (stale) or canned food or food cooked in microwave. Always listen to Dr. Leo Rebello. If he is not around, consult your grand mother, for she is certainly wiser than all the so-called medical experts who know more and more of less and less.

KALA-AZAR

Kala-azar means black water sickness or black fever. The terms originally referred to Indian *visceral leishmaniasis,* due to its characteristic symptoms, blackening or darkening of the skin of the hands, feet, face and the abdomen (Lainson and Shaw, 1987). It is also called leishmaniasis and tropical splenomegaly (since spleen enlarges bigger than the liver).

Cutaneous leishmaniasis causes skin sores, and *visceral leishmaniasis (VL),* affects some of the internal organs of the body, for example, spleen, liver, bone marrow. People who have VL usually have fever, weight loss; show low blood counts, including low RBCs, WBCs and platelet count.

Leishmaniasis is found in about 88 tropical and subtropical countries from rain forests in Central and South America to deserts in West Asia. More than 90 percent of the world's cases of VL are in Bangladesh, Brazil, India, Nepal and Sudan.

It is spread by the bite of sand flies which become infected by biting an infected animal (for example, a rodent or dog) or person. Since sand flies are small and do not make noise when they fly, people may not realize they are present. They are usually active from dusk to dawn.

However, they will bite if they are disturbed, such as when a person brushes up against the trunk of a tree where sand flies are resting. *Kala-azar* can also be spread by blood transfusions or contaminated needles. Adventure travelers, Peace Corps volunteers, missionaries, ornithologists and people who work outdoors at night, tribals who do not have adequate clothes, and soldiers are examples of people who may have an increased risk for *Kala-azar.*

Diagnosing *Kala-azar* can be difficult. Sometimes the laboratory tests are negative even if a person has leishmaniasis. If you are not sleeping in an area that is well screened or air-conditioned, use a bed net and tuck it under the mattress. If possible, use a bed net that has been soaked in or sprayed with *permethrin,* which will be effective for several months if the bed net is not washed.

VL is caused by the parasites *Leishmania donovani donovani, Leishmania donovani infantum, Leishmania donovani archibaldi* and *Leishmania donovani chagasi.* In endemic cases of VL, the disease is chronic and onset is gradual. Although people of all ages are susceptible, children below the age of 15 are more commonly affected with *L.d infantum* being largely responsible (*Rab et al*, 1995).

The common symptoms of VL include high undulating fever often with two or even three peaks in 24 hours and drenching sweats, chills, rigors, weight loss, fatigue and poor appetite, cough, burning feet, insomnia, abdominal pain, joint pain, anorexia, epistaxis and diarrhoea. Clinical signs include splenomegaly, hepatomegaly and lymphadenopathy (Hashim *et al*, 1994). The incubation period is highly variable, between ten days to over a year. The duration of the disease can be 1-20 weeks, in endemic areas of Western Sudan the illness usually lasts about 12-16 weeks with an average of about 6 weeks.

VL can be complicated by serious secondary infections such as pneumonia, dysentery and pulmonary tuberculosis, which often contribute to the high fatality rate of VL patients. Other complications though rare include haemolytic anemia, acute renal damage and severe mucosal haemorrhage (WHO expert committee report, 1991).

Post *Kala-azar* dermal leishmaniasis (PKDL) occurs in India, Sudan, Kenya, China and Iraq. The disease begins with small lesions (hypopigmented macules, papules or nodules) appearing on the face (rarely greater than 1cm in diameter). Eventually the lesions spread to the upper trunk, arms, forearms, thighs, legs, abdomen, the neck and the back. The multiple lesions can coalesce to form larger lesions and lead to the gross enlargement of facial features such as the nose and lips, giving an appearance similar to leprosy. The disease is particularly severe if the lesions spread to the mucosal surfaces of the nasal septum, hard and soft palate, oropharynx, larynx or the eye lids and the cornea leading to blindness (Hashim and Ramesh *et al*, 1995). Lesions can also occur on the glans of the penis and genital mucosa.

Hence, the possibility of PKDL being transmitted sexually. In addition to the disease being confused with leprosy, PKDL can also resemble secondary syphillis and sarcoidosis. The lesions are usually self-limiting; however those that do not heal within six months should be treated.

Pentavalent antimonials remain the drugs of choice for treating PKDL. *Sodium stibogluconate* at a dose of 20 mg/kg of body weight administered intramuscularly for 4-5 months is recommended. In addition *Ketoconazole* and *allopurinol* can be given orally to improve response. In antimony resistant cases *amphotericin B* is an effective replacement (Ramesh *et al*, 1995). Clarke in his Prescriber says that Antimony is the antidote to *Kala-azar.* It is injected intravenously in the form of *Stibacetin* beginning with 0.1 grm. and working up generally to 0.8 grm. Or a colloidal preparation of *Oxide of Antimony* may be injected intra-muscularly (1 - 50th of a grain in 15 drops of *Glycerine* and 15 drops of distilled water).

Homeopathic remedies for Kala-azar are:

Antimonium crudum, Antim metallicum or Antim tart: Indicated in bilharzia, sleeping sickness, oriental boils, kala-azar and venereal granuloma. *Arsenicum album:* Infantile kala-azar (Dr. Neatby). Spleen enlarged, great debility, exhaustion, restlessness, with nightly aggravation; skin like parchment. *Ferrum arsenicosum:* Enlarged liver and spleen with fever, diarrhoea, undigested stool, clammy sweat, and staining linen yellow, restless at night in bed. *Natrum muriaticum:* Intermittent fever, anemia, great debility, most weak in the morning, coldness of body and continuous chilliness.

In Ayurveda, *Vitex Penduncularis* is used as a substitute for quinine. A short time after its administration the patient's blood is found to be entirely free from malaria germs, *kala-azar* and haemoglobinuric fever. It is a non-toxic, non-depressant and a safe drug. It has no bitter taste. Infusion of leaves, root bark or young stem is used several times a day by the aboriginal tribes of Bihar and Orissa for malaria and black water fevers.

LEPROSY

Leprosy (Hansen's disease) has been known since biblical times. It is characterized by disfiguring skin lesions, peripheral nerve damage, progressive debilitation and cosmetic disfigurement. It has a long incubation period (3 to 5 years) and children are more susceptible to it. There are broadly two types of leprosy - *lepramatous,* in which the damage is more widespread, progressive and severe; and *tubercular,* which is milder. Contrary to popular belief, it is not highly contagious. Hence, isolation of victims in 'leper colonies' is unnecessary.

Leprosy is caused by *Mycobacterium leprae,* spread through droplets of nasal mucus. A person is infectious to others only during the first stages of the disease and only people living in prolonged close contact with an infected person are at risk of contracting it.

Initially, damage is confined to peripheral nerves, which supply the skin and muscles. Skin areas supplied by affected nerves become lighter or darker and sensation / sweating in these areas are reduced. As the disease progresses, the peripheral nerves swell and become tender. Hands, feet and facial skin eventually become numb and muscles become paralysed. Complications include loss of all sensation in the hands and feet, so that accidental burns or injuries are not noticed, leading to extensive scarring or even loss of fingers or toes. Muscle paralysis can lead to further deformity.

Damage to the facial nerve means that the eyelids cannot be closed, the cornea dries, leading to inflammation and ulceration of the eyeball and blindness. The disability caused by the combined effects of blindness and loss of touch sensation is extremely severe. Cartilage and bone in the nose are often eroded, and bones elsewhere in the body may be weakened. The testes may atrophy leading to sterility.

Leprosy is common in temperate, tropical, and subtropical climates. Worldwide, there are about 20 million sufferers (about 2 million permanently disabled). Brazil, Madagascar, Mozambique, Tanzania and Nepal together account for 90% cases.

Early diagnosis is essential to prevent permanent disfigurement and disability. A provisional diagnosis is made from the skin patch appearing on the body. This patch shifts from one place to another and hence it is called 'butterfly patch'. It is small, has a ring around it and a pin prick inside the ring will not give any sensation. Skin biopsy is a confirmatory test.

In Allopathy, a combination of Dapsone, Rifampin and Clofazimine is used that kills most of the causative bacteria within a few days, it is claimed. And yet they will say that these medicines should be taken for over a period of two years or for lifetime. Other medicines like ethionamide, aspirin, prednisone, or thalidomide are used for the control of inflammation (e.g. *erythema nodosum leprosum*). This has led to the emergence of drug-resistant *Mycobacterium leprae*, as well as increased numbers of cases worldwide, indicating once again that modern medicine's business model of treating disease is failing. Yet they go on hoodwinking people *ad nauseam*.

Homeopathy is very effective in Leprosy. The medicines are:
Alumina: Leprous pimples, scurf and tetters, which itch or become moist chiefly in the evening. *Anacardium occidentale (cashew nut):* Anaesthetic variety of leprosy. *Antimonium tartaricum:* Heaviness in limbs followed by leprous eruption; small ulcers on tips of fingers and toes, spreading, livid edges. *Arsenicum album:* yellow or white spots; tubercular swelling in the nose; burning ulcers at the ends of the fingers, at the toes, soles of feet, navel and cheek; raised up tubercles; hyperæsthesia and anæsthesia alternating. *Asimina triloba (custard apple):* Tubercular leprosy. *Calotropis gigantea* - In lupus of face, thickening of the skin; heals the ulcers and blotches from the skin and perfects the cure. *Causticum:* Foot feels contracted, with tension on putting it to the ground; numbness of feet and toes. *Graphites:* Leprous spots, coppery, annular, raised on face, ears, buttocks, legs and feet; ulcers on toes, obduration of nose, crusts in nostrils. *Hydrastis canadensis:* Indicated during the ulcerative stage, when it meets the secondary symptoms, the lowered vitality and impaired constitutional effects. *Hydrocotyle asiatica:* Has considerable reputation in leprosy and lupus, when there is no ulceration. It has ameliorated cases of leprosy, arrested the destructive process. *Phosphorus:* Leprosy, later stages; brown spots on an even base; tubercles on trunk and buttocks; thick patches on face and arms; tension in fingers and dullness towards the ends.

Piper methysticum: Skin is covered with large scales, which fall off leaving white spots, and these often become ulcers. Dryness, especially where it is thick, as on hands and feet, with scales. *Psorinum (sero-purulent matter of scabies nosode):* Clarke indicates this nosode in leprosy. *Secale cornutum:* According to Bhanja, it is the principal remedy for leprosy.

Neem Oil produced from the seed of ripe fruits from Neem *(Azadirachta Indica)* tree cures leprosy, eczema and some other obstinate skin diseases. Neem leaves can also be eaten and Neem juice enema will cleanse the intestines. Charak also recommends *Boerhavia diffusa (Punarnabha, Spreading Hog-wide)* and *Caesalpinia bonducella (Fever nut)* in leprosy. *Chaulmoogra (Taraktogenos)* is also effective in early stages.

The vegetables and fruits most suitable in Leprosy: Cabbage, cauliflower, black currants, grapes, mangoes, yellow bananas, yellow pumpkin may be consumed a lot. These contain the natural sulphur, phenols which disinfect and clean the system. Buttermilk and curd should be consumed daily between 11 am and 2 pm. Apply Turmeric paste on the affected parts and expose the affected parts to the morning sun for about 10 minutes. Yoga posture Sarvangasan is specific in leprosy. Suryanamaskar will tone up the entire body. Sulphur tub bath, mud bath also give very good results. Sleeping in the solarium with yellow cellophane will filter golden rays on the body, which will heal the body, mind and the spirit fully.

MALARIA

Malaria is spread by *Anopheles mosquitoes*. The disease produces severe fever and, in some cases, complications affecting the kidneys, liver, brain and blood which can be fatal.

Malaria is prevalent throughout the tropics, affecting upto 500 million people worldwide each year. Malaria kills about one million children every year in Africa alone.

The WHO has undertaken a massive programme of malaria control, but little progress has been made in the past 25 years. Mosquitoes have developed resistance to insecticides and anti-malarial drugs.

The parasites responsible for malaria are protozoa known as plasmodia. Four species can cause disease in humans, namely, *Plasmodium falciparum, P.vivax, P.ovale and P.malariae.* The parasites grow in the liver of a person for a few days and then enter the bloodstream where they invade the red blood cells.

The period between being bitten by the mosquito and the appearance of the symptoms is usually a week or two. Symptoms include shaking chills and fever, which appear only when RBCs that are infected with parasites rupture to release more parasites into the blood stream. The principal symptom of infection is the classical malarial ague. Usually the fever has three stages: a cold stage of rigors (uncontrollable shivering); a hot stage in which the temperature may reach alarmingly high and finally a sweating stage that drenches the bedding and brings down the body temperature. A severe headache, general malaise and vomiting may accompany the attack. At the end of an attack the patient is left weak and tired and sleeps.

P.falciparum infects all RBCs, whereas the other varieties attack only young or old cells. This fever can be more fatal, as the affected RBCs become sticky and block blood vessels in vital organs, especially the kidneys. The spleen becomes enlarged and the brain may be affected, leading to convulsions and coma. Destruction of blood cells leads to haemolytic anaemia, kidney failure and jaundice.

Malaria parasites can be identified by examining under the microscope a drop of the patient's blood. Other methods are: **(a)** Antigen detection in which kits of rapid diagnostic tests are used. Such immuno-chromatographic tests provide results in 2-10 minutes. **(b)** Molecular diagnosis using polymerase chain reaction. This technique is more accurate. But, it is expensive and requires a specialized laboratory. **(c)** Serology detects antibodies against malaria parasites, using either indirect immunofluorescence or enzyme-linked immunosorbent assay (ELISA). Serology does not detect current infection. In *P. falciparum* malaria, additional laboratory findings may include mild anemia, decrease in blood platelets (thrombocytopenia), elevation of bilirubin, aminotransferases, albuminuria, and the presence of abnormal bodies in the urine (urinary casts).

In severe cases of *falciparum* malaria, doctors may give you *blood transfusions* along with drugs. We have heard of 'double jeopardy' (a legal expression meaning double punishment). But here it is triple punishment.

You suffer due to malaria, and then you are given strong drugs that give you 'iatrogenic disorders', and blood transfusions which may transfer someone else's diseases to you.

Chloroquine, which is said to eradicate malaria from the blood, is the usual treatment for all types of malaria. *Quinine* is used where chloroquine fails. Patients suffering from *vivax* or *ovale* are also prescribed *primaquine* to eradicate parasites in the liver. *Primaquine* may cause *haemolytic anaemia* in people suffering from *G6PD deficiency.* The other drugs that are used include *proguanil, pyrimethamine* and *dapsone.*

According to the Complete Health Encyclopedia of the British Medical Association, "Even people who take antimalarial drugs and precautions against bites may contract malaria".

The real cause of infectious disease is wrong feeding habits and faulty life-style, resulting in the system being clogged with morbid matter. The liberal use of denatured foods of today like KFC, Big Mac, mugs-full of coffee and beers, cokes and drugging the system right from mother's womb, weakens the system and paves the way for the development of diseases, over which the pharma-mafia thrives. The entire edifice of modern medicine is unscientific and rotten to the core.

Treatment: Diet, as I have emphasized all along, is of utmost importance in the treatment of any disease. The patient should fast on diluted orange juice for five to ten days, depending on the severity of malaria to remove toxins, acids from the intestine and liver and to alkalize the blood. To bring the fever down, full body compresses, sponging the body, sitz baths, and enemas are indicated. If there are chills, warm water enema, if there is fever, cold water enema. After the fever has gone, the patient may be put on fruit diet, consisting of fruits like oranges, grapes, grape-fruit, apple, pineapple, mango and papaya. Fresh curds may be added to the diet after about three days of fruit diet. Cinnamon with pepper and honey is very effective in malaria. Infusion of the leaves of holy basil (*tulsi*) and neem can also be used.

Homeopathy has several remedies for Malaria. But China, China sulph, Arsenic album and Natrum muriaticum would head the list. Lower potencies work better in Malaria.

China officinalis (Peruvian or Cinchona Bark): The paroxysm is preceded by headache, nausea, hunger, anguish and palpitation of the heart. Thirst before the chill and during the sweating stage. Chills alternating with heat, skin cold and blue, headache, nausea and absence of thirst. During hot stage, dryness of the mouth and lips, red face and headache. After the heat, thirst and profuse sweat. Ringing in the ears, with dizziness and a feeling as if the head was enlarged. Pain in the region of the liver and spleen when bending or coughing. *This was the first Homeopathic remedy discovered by Hahnemann to cure Malaria.*

Chininum sulphuricum (Sulphate of Quinine): Acute malaria. The patient is exhausted and there is constant ringing in the ears and vertigo occurring periodically, with chills and fever; cerebral congestion and partial deafness.

Cornus circinata: Chronic malarial troubles, with jaundice, tendency to diarrhoea or dysentery, congested liver, enlarged spleen, etc.

Arsenicum album: Usual time of aggravation is 1 to 2 p.m. or 12 to 2 a.m. Unquenchable thirst for large quantities of cold water, with vomiting after drinking. Tongue is furred on the sides, with red streak down the middle. Enlargement and induration of the liver and spleen following malaria. According to Grimmer, on getting into the infected territory a dose of Arsenic album 30th potency to be taken once a week for a month.

Natrium muriaticum: Intermittent fever, chill beginning at 10 a.m., with thirst, pains, profuse sweat relieving all symptoms; throbbing frontal headache generally accompanies the chill and fever. It is useful in chronic malarial conditions with weakness, constipation, and loss of appetite in those who have taken much quinine. According to Grimmer, as a preventive, one should have a dose of Nat-m. 30 or higher once a week, for four to six weeks when visiting/working in mosquitoes infested areas.

Malaria officinalis (Malaria Nosode, decomposed vegetable matter): Has evident power to cause the disappearance of the plasmodium of malaria. Malarial cachexia. Spleen affections. Malaria and rheumatism. According to Kamthan, one dose of the 200th potency per week is sufficient.

The other Homeopathic remedies in Alphabetical order are:

Alstonia constricta: The bark of this tree enjoys great repute in India for the cure of malarial diseases, diarrhoea and dysentery with debility and malarial anaemia. Used as a tonic after exhausting malaria, 5-drop dose in cold water after meals.

Aranea diadema: Great regularity of paroxysm, at precisely same hour, every day, or every other day. Chilliness not relieved by anything, with pains in long bones. For those who are suffering from the chronic effects of malarial poisoning, or who live in damp, wet places. Reduces enlarged spleen.

Arnica montana: Indicated in cases maltreated with Quinine than any other remedy; and here lies its chief value in the treatment of intermittent fever.

Boletus laricis: Loss of appetite; pale and anaemic from chronic malaria.

Cactus grandiflorus: Haemorrhage from the bowels in malarial fevers.

Caesalpinia bonducella: Irregular and shivering fever, on alternate days; burning sensation of the limbs; Malaria or Black-fever; the face turns pale during fever; fever from 6 pm to 10 pm.

Capsicum annuum (Cayenne Pepper): Bursting headache with malaria, liver and spleen are enlarged, especially if the spleen is sensitive, swollen, indurated. In the acute cases the chill begins in the back, between the scapulae or in the lumbar region. There is great thirst during the chill and every drink is followed by a shudder.

Cedron: It has proved curative in marsh malaria characterized by severe pains recurring periodically, with enlarged spleen and liver, general anaemia and dropsy. Often there is regular recurrence of supra-orbital neuralgia with the fever.

Crotalus horridus (remedy prepared from the poison of rattlesnake): Malaria with exhausted vital force. Haemorrhages, blood flows from eyes, ears, nose, and every orifice of the body. Haemolytic jaundice.

Eucalyptus globulus: The remedy is indicated in sub-acute and chronic malarial infectious cases, in which large quantities of quinine have been employed.

Gelsemium (Yellow Jasmine): periodic fever, generally coming on towards evening, with stupor, dizziness, blindness, faintness, no thirst, great prostration, slight perspiration, which relieves. Eyelids heavy.

Gentiana Chirata (Indian Gentian, Chirata): gives excellent result in Malaria, Influenza and Typhoid etc.

Ipecac: When there is any doubt in regard to the choice of a remedy, especially at the commencement of the disease, this remedy may be administered.

Lycopodium: Chronic malarial fever, paroxysms recurring at 4 p.m., there is general nervous irritability, with thirst, red sand in the urine, enlargement of spleen, sour vomiting between chill and heat, teasing cough, the chill often beginning in the back.

Parthenium hysterophorus: This remedy and its alkaloid is employed in the relief of malarial fever in the tropics of Cuba and Panama. It has not only controlled the early attack, but has reduced the enlarged liver and spleen, which are painful to the touch. It has controlled the periodical neuralgia that attends many of these cases after quinine has failed.

Podophyllum: a curative remedy in chronic relapsing malarial fever, to be given in 1M potency.

Terebinthiniae oleum: recommended as a prophylactic in malarial fevers.

Vitex negundo: Used in the Andamans in Mother Tincture for treatment of Malaria.

Biochemic remedies for Malaria are: Ferrum phosphoricum 6X, Kali muriaticum 6X, Natrum sulphuricum 6X – 2 to 4 tablets, per dose, in alternation with any one of the indicated Homeopathic remedies

RABIES

Rabies is an acute viral disease of the central nervous system (CNS). It was formerly known as hydrophobia. According to medical literature, it is 100% fatal once symptoms develop. But such a scare is un-called for; because fear can paralyse or kill a person (refer to *psycho-neuro-immunology* of a disease), like more people die due to fright of snake bite rather than the snake bite, *per se*.

Except for Australia and Antartic regions, rabies is spread throughout the world. Rabies primarily affects animals, but it can be transmitted from a rabid animal to a human by a bite or by a lick over a break in the skin. The causative virus, present in the animal's saliva, travels from the wound along nerve pathways to the brain. The incubation period between a bite and the appearance of symptoms is between nine days and eight weeks, depending largely on the size and depth of the bite, and proximity to the CNS. The first symptoms are fever, headache and loss of appetite, leading to restlessness, hyperactivity, disorientation, and, in some cases, seizures.

Often the victim is intensely thirsty, but attempts to drink induce violent, painful spasms in the throat (hence the term hydrophobia). Eye and facial muscles may become paralysed. Encephalitis, coma and death follow within three to twenty days after the onset of symptoms, if not treated properly and timely.

A Manual of Materia Medica Therapeutics and Pharmacy by A.L. Blackwood lists the symptoms of Rabies as under:

The first symptom noticed is a slight difficulty in swallowing, accompanied by nervousness and irritability. Hyperaesthesia develops rapidly, until in a few hours, a slight noise or the sight of anything bright and shining brings on a convulsion. The pulse is very rapid, the respiration spasmodic and jerky.

This spasmodic condition attacks the throat in particular, and any attempt to swallow, especially water, causes a convulsive closure of the pharynx, although the patient is usually extremely thirsty. The condition eventually becomes so acute that the sight or even the thought of water brings on a paroxysm. Hallucinations usually accompany this stage of the disease, and at times violent mania develops. Later the excitement gives way to collapse; the patient becomes relaxed and quiet, and finally lapses into unconsciousness.

Most human cases result from a bite by a rabid dog. The rabid dog can be identified thus: It barks for a long period, snarls, has a ferocious look, saliva dribbles from its mouth, it goes round and round, runs after animals and vehicles and attacks without provocation.

Allopathy treats the symptoms with sedative and analgesic drugs (painkillers) which aggravates the condition of the patient. If there is a risk of rabies, passive immunization is given with human rabies immunoglobulin (ready-made antibodies against the rabies virus), and rabies vaccine is given by a course of injections lasting several weeks along with anti-tetanus. If a healthy animal remains symptom-free after five days, treatment of the bitten person is stopped. If immunization is given within two days of the bite, rabies is almost always prevented, it is claimed.

Most rabies viruses belong to genus Lyssavirus and the family Rhabdoviridae. Rabies is spread through the bite wound (80% cases) or contact with saliva of the infected animals. Exposures involving small rodents and lagomorphs (eg, squirrels, hamsters, guinea pigs, gerbils, chipmunks, rats, mice, rabbits, hares) do not require treatment. These animals can be infected with rabies virus in the lab but have never been associated with transmission to humans.

But bites or scratches from high-risk animals, such as bats, raccoons, foxes, skunks, woodchucks, and nondomestic dogs should be immediately treated.

Direct human-to-human transmission of rabies has not been documented. However, six cases have been reported in which people died of rabies after transplantation of corneas from people who were diagnosed with the disease.

WHO estimates that about 35,000 die worldover from rabies annually. That is a very, very small number. But the business of medicine must go on. So, the allopath will ask you to do costly, time consuming and dangerous Lab Studies consisting of lumbar puncture and taking your cerebrospinal fluid (CSF) even though it may be negative for seven days even after clinical illness has begun. They will also do what they call "definitive diagnosis" of detection of direct fluorescent antibody from the brain or nerves surrounding hair follicles in the nape of neck, in addition to isolating the rabies virus from saliva, and skin biopsy to detect rabies antigen in hair follicles. They will then do your head CT scan though everything will show normal. Finally, when you die due to their mistakes, they will do postmortem and find Negri bodies in the hippocampus and Purkinje cells of the cerebellum. "These are found in 70-80% of cases along with perivascular inflammation of gray matter", they will conclude.

The three rabies vaccines currently available are the human diploid cell vaccine (HDCV, Imovax), rabies vaccine adsorbed (RVA), and RabAvert (rabies vaccine produced by Chiron). They are equal in efficacy and safety, it is claimed.

The vaccine takes 7-10 days to induce an active immune response, with immunity lasting approximately two years. They are administered in the deltoid region, with a dose of 1 mL on days 0, 3, 7, 14, and 28.

Contraindications: Slight erythema, hyper-sensitivity and anaphylactic reactions may occur. Caution is indicated in thrombocytopenia or bleeding disorders. Safety of these vaccines, for use during pregnancy, has not been established. Also, those on corticosteroids, antimalarials, and other immunosuppressive agents may not benefit.

Rest the patient, counsel him or her, wash the wound with salt or sour lime, or potassium permanganate and bandage the wound lightly with homeopathic ledum, hypericum and calendula mother tinctures. For one week put the patient on fruit juices, and let the patient take homeopathic prophylactic like *Hydrophobinum, Lyssinum, Curare* and other homeopathic medicines, if required.

In India, the villagers use *Cerebera odollam* fruit with *Datura Fastuosa* (thorn apple) seeds for hydrophobia. Likewise, *Ophiorrhiza mungos* (mongoose plant) is used as an antidote against the bites of mad dogs. The drug is an agreeable bitter tonic.

Homeopathic Remedy, *Lyssinum* is specific and also prophylactic. *Lyssinum* is a trituration of sugar of milk saturated with the saliva of a rabid dog. Symptoms include dread of liquids; profuse salivation; swelling of the mouth; intense frontal headache; trembling; convulsions with periodic spasms; stiffness and coldness; the same kind of nerve irritation as caused by the poison of rabies. Used to remove the bad-effects of anti-rabies vaccination. According to Dr. Kent, it takes the pain out of a dog bite. It takes the fear from the patient.

The other remedies indicated are: *Agave americana* for hydrophobia. *Belladonna:* in encephalitis, the suffocation caused by drinking with inordinate thirst, the general inability to swallow anything, the desire to bite those around him alternating with terror; answers to Blackwood symptoms of Rabies listed above. It is one of Boenninghausen's Rabies powders.

Curare (a South American arrow poison): said to be an antidote to the rabies poison. *Euphorbia splendida:* recommended much in rabies canina as tincture or infusum. *Hyosyamus niger:* for hydrophobia and also listed as a prophylactic. Boenninghausen recommends this too. *Stramonium:* Another of Boenninghausen's Rabies powders. Delirium, screaming and howling in a high voice.

Tanacetum vulgare: induces all the cardinal features of rabies : convulsions, frothy, bloody mucus in the air passages, hallucinations, convulsions without loss of consciousness, opisthotonos, spasms of pharynx, larynx, and thorax, abundant salivation, sensual excitability, tendency to bite, hoarse cry, diminished sensibility and mobility, momentary paralysis, sub-pleural ecchymoses, infarctions of the liver.

Viscum album (Mistletoe): According to Laville, all mistletoes are useful in epilepsy and rabies..

TUBERCULOSIS

Tuberculosis (also known as consumption or phthisis) is a wasting disease caused by a slow-growing aerobic bacterium, *Mycobacterium tuberculosis*. It is spread through cough, sneeze, speak, or spit of the active TB patient. Close contacts (spouse, child, health care worker) can be affected.

Tuberculosis mainly affects lungs, intestines, bones and glands. Pulmonary or lung TB is the commonest (75 to 80 percent). Symptoms are prolonged cough of more than three weeks duration, chest pain, and hemoptysis. Also, fever, chills, night sweats, appetite loss, weight loss, and easy fatigability.

Other sites include the pleura, central nervous system (meningitis), lymphatic system (scrofula of the neck), genitourinary system, and bones and joints (Pott's disease of the spine). An especially serious form is *disseminated* or *miliary* TB, so named because the lung lesions so-formed resemble millet seeds on x-ray. These are more common in immuno-suppressed persons and in young children.

Low immunity increases the risk of progression to TB disease. For example, substance abuse, more particularly I.V. drug use, diabetes mellitus, silicosis, prolonged corticosteroid therapy and other immunosuppressive therapy, intestinal bypass or gastrectomy, chronic malabsorption syndromes, or low body weight. Some drugs, like rheumatoid arthritis drugs that work by blocking the tumor necrosis factor-alpha (an inflammation-causing cytokine), raise the risk of causing a latent infection to become active.

Medical evaluation for TB includes a medical history, a physical examination, a tuberculin skin test, a chest X-ray, and microbiologic smears and cultures.

Lowered resistance or devitalisation of the system is the chief cause of this disease. Other causes include exposure to cold, loss of sleep, impure air, a sedentary life, exhausting work, disorders of digestion and assimilation, impoverishment of the blood due to malnutrition, improper treatment of other diseases, depressing mental emotions, use of tobacco in any form, liquor, coffee etc. and anything that lowers the vital force.

There are only four known cures for consumption: the rest cure, the food cure, the air cure and the mind cure. Fresh air, sun baths, special exercises for developing the muscles of the chest can be recommended. In Yoga we have chest capacity building, colon cleansing, oxygenation and relaxation exercises.

Vegetables like drumstick, snake gourd, spinach and *methi* (fenugreek), in particular, are very good, as also no phlegm forming fruits. No banana, guava, lady's finger are to be taken. Likewise, milk is contraindicated in TB. Plenty of grapes should be eaten to cleanse up the blood. Wheat Grass, sprouts, carrots and radish, in particular, will tone up the body faster. Custard apple is considered specific.

Ayurvedic practitioners use *Sitaphalasava* which is available with Ayurvedic chemists in India. Others can prepare the decoction by boiling custard apple *(Sitaphal)* pulp and seedless raisins in water on slow fire. Filter it when about one third water is left. Then mix it with powdered sugar candy and also the powders of cardamom, cinnamon and slight turmeric. Fresh *Aamla* (indian gooseberry) juice, one tablespoonful mixed with honey given first thing in the morning is very beneficial. Within a few days the TB patient will get strength.

Also note this simple home remedy: 30 grams of garlic to be boiled in 16 tablespoons of milk and about 3 cups of water. After boiling reduce to one-fourth quantity and filter. Give this to the patient twice daily till the mucous from the lungs clears.

Homeopathy - Over a hundred homeopathic remedies are indicated in tuberculosis. However, since TB is a constitutional disease, it is of paramount importance to administer the proper constitutional remedy, rather than one directed to the isolated symptoms.

Arsenicum iodatum (Iodide of Arsenic) is a very-near specific in TB. Pulmonary tuberculosis, with cavities in lungs, profound prostration, rapid, irritable pulse, recurring fever and sweats, tendency to diarrhea. Clinically, it has been found advisable in tuberculosis to begin with about the 4x and gradually go lower to the 2x trituration, 3 times a day.

Another specific is: *Acalypha indica (Indian Nettle).* Tubercular deposits in apex of lung leading to cough with bloody expectoration.

There are also nosodes like *Bacillinum* (a maceration of a typical tuberculous lung) and *Tuberculinum* (prepared from tubercular abscess). These are more effective than BCG and without its side effects.

Bacillinum: Works to ameliorate the symptoms of lung TB. Less thick sputum, the cavities are drier, less congestion, less cough and less expectoration. Patient tends to put on weight and on the way to recovery with proper food in less than three months. *Tuberculinum bovinum (a nosode from tubercular abscess):* Clears opacities from old tubercular corneitis and helps in tubercular meningitis, with effusion. Arrests further progress of the disease. It often gives immunity if taken before the tuberculosis begins in those who have inherited it.

Glands: Carboneum Sulph, Bacillinum, Kali-iod., Drosera, Ars Iod, Calcarea Iod, Tuberculinum bov. **Lungs:** Especially Acalypha indica, Ars iod. **Intestines:** Ferrum aceticum, Ars iod, Abrotanum, Calcarea carb, Calcarea phos, Iodum, Calcarea hypophos. **Bones:** Drosera, Calc. carb., Calcarea hypophos, Calc phos, Hepar sulph., Mezereum, Phosphorus, Pulsatilla, Radium Brom, Silicea, Tuberculinum bov.

Other Homeopathic Medicines indicated in Tuberculosis Are:
Apis mellifica (Poison of the Honey Bee)**:** In meningitis, acute or chronic, or tubercular hydrocephalus, the child bores the head into the pillow. *Bromium***:** is indicated in tuberculosis of the lungs, particularly the right lung. The patient suffers frequently from congestion of the head and chest, which is relieved by nose-bleed. Stony, hard, scrofulous or tuberculous swelling of glands, especially on lower jaw and throat. *Calcarea hypophosphorosa* **:** Indicated in Mesenteric TB, hectic fever, night sweats,

haemoptysis and profuse menstruation in the female. *Cannabis Sativa* (Hemp): Zopfy based on his 60 years experience recommends *Kali hydroiodicum* and *Cannabis sativa* in tuberculosis. He used the 1x of each in alternation, and concludes that no remedies in the entire Materia Medica have such an influence in lessening the cough, the expectoration, the colliquative sweats and the hectic fever. *Carboneum sulphuratum* : Tubercular affections of larynx, glands, testes and ovaries. *Drosera rotundifolia* : It raises the resistance against tuberculosis. Hahnemann considered it the only remedy in laryngeal phthisis. Also effective in tubercular glands and TB of bones, lungs and larynx. *Helleborus niger* (Christmas Rose): Tubercular hydrocephalus, which develops rapidly, automatic motion of one arm and leg. *Lachesis mutus* (Surucucu Snake poison): Tuberculosis following pneumonia. *Lecithinum* (Phosphorus-containing complex organic body prepared from the yolk of egg and animal brains): TB of the young, they are tired, weak and complain of a loss of flesh, short breath and general exhaustion. *Natrium sulphuricum* : Abdominal tuberculosis, chronic diarrhea. *Nitricum acidum* (Nitric acid): A powerful anti-tubercular remedy before cavities are formed. Most useful in phthisis of young girls. *Rumex crispus* : Advanced state of tuberculosis: cough worse from talking; sharp stitching pains through left lung; passes urine or stool with violent cough. *Tarentula cubensis* (Cuban Spider): Produces euthanasia in the last days of pulmonary TB patients; soothes the agony of death. *Thuja occidentalis* (Tree of Life; White Cedar): In far-advanced tuberculosis of the lungs a dose of Thuja gives great relief, by the evacuation of large masses of pus, by means of cough, diminishes the night sweats, and restores the lost appetite.

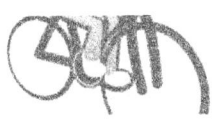

TYPHOID

Typhoid fever is a bacterial infection of the intestinal tract and occasionally the bloodstream. It is also called Enteric Fever and is caused through *Salmonella typhi*, passed through faeces or urine of the infected person mixed in food and water due to poor hygiene.

Early symptoms: fever, malaise, abdominal pain, headache, constipation alternated with diarrhea, rose-coloured spots on chest and abdomen and an enlarged spleen and liver. The tongue is coated, there may be bleeding from the nose. In the second week high fever is prevalent along with trembling and delirium. Pulse is relatively low. Weakness, profound fatigue, delirium, and an acutely ill appearance develops. Complications can be intestinal hemorrhage (severe GI bleeding), intestinal perforation, kidney failure and peritonitis.

Typhoid begins like a cold and then temperature increases day by day. The fever is at its peak on the 8th day. There is headache and sore throat, tired feeling and frequent chills.

Allopaths will ask you to do following tests, while you burn with fever:
· An elevated white blood cell count in blood.
· A blood culture during first week of the fever to show *S. typhi* bacteria.
· A stool culture.
· An Elisa test on urine that may show Vi antigen specific for the bacteria
· A platelet count (to show decreased platelets).
· A fluorescent antibody study (demonstrating Vi antigen, specific for typhoid).

Allopathic treatment consists of antibiotics, such as, chloramphenicol, ampicillin or ciprofloxacin. There are increasing rates of antibiotic resistance throughout the world, so the choice of antibiotics should be a careful one.

Intravenous fluids and electrolytes will be routinely administered in allopathic hospitals along with antibiotics, stronger antibiotics making simple disease more complicated.

One thumb rule: For any fever which lasts more than 5 days, the person should go on only a fruit juice, milk and water fast. Salads such as cabbage

58

and carrots can be taken. Cooked food should not be taken except watery vegetable soups as one should not burden the intestines in enteric fever. Jejube berries, raisins and sugar candy (*mishri*) in the ratio 2:3:1 should be taken after boiling in about 100ml of water and strained. The decoction should be taken in small doses if rash appears.

Constipation should not be allowed to develop and the person should drink lots of water and have watery fruits like orange or citric juices diluted with water. Lower the fever with cold compresses on the abdomen. It may also be applied if the person defecates blood, has unbearable pain in the intestines which may be due to bowel perforation.

Do not eat food exposed to flies especially during fairs, festivals and rainy season. Always boil the drinking water. The person having typhoid should be isolated. Dishes, clothes of that person should not be shared. Person nursing a typhoid patient should maintain utmost hygiene.

Typhoid vaccine is available, but it is neither safe nor sound to take it before traveling. As long as you pay strict attention to food and water you should be fine. Homeopathic nosode called *Typhoidinum* can be taken during typhoid epidemic as prophylactic or as a first remedy when first indication of internal derangement manifests. Take *Typhoidinum 1M/4 pills* before travel and be carefree, but not careless.

Baptisia tinctoria (Wild Indigo), *Pyrogen* (artificial Sepsin) could be considered somewhat specific homeopathic remedies. *Veratrum viride* (Green Hellebore) is also very effective in typhoid fever, with blood dysentery and black lumps.

For the prodrome, based on symptoms and to prevent the disease from progressing, remedies like Gelsemium, Baptisia, Bryonia, Rhus tox will be much useful. For the stage after the prodrome, in addition to the above mentioned remedies, Lachesis, Phosphoric acid, Arnica, may be indicated. For advanced stages, Lycopodium, Carbo veg, Muriatic acid, Opium may be required.

Biochemic remedies in 6x potency for Typhoid are:

Calcarea phosphoricum (phosphate of Lime): After typhoid, as the disease declines. *Ferrum phosphoricum (phosphate of Iron):* During the beginning of typhoid fevers. High fever, quick pulse and increased temperature; copious night-sweats; dry heat of palms, face, throat and chest. *Kali muriaticum (potassium chloride):* looseness of bowels, flocculent evacuations with grey-white coated tongue. Suits the second stage of disease. *Kali phosphoricum (potassium phosphate):* For haemorrhages in typhoid, septic states, offensive, carrion-like diarrhea, brown, dry tongue, petechiae, sleeplessness, stupor, delirium. *Kali sulphuricum (Glauber's salt, potassium sulphate):* Typhoid, with rise of temperature at night and fall in the morning. *Natrum muriaticum (common salt, sodium chloride):* Typhoid with twitchings, drowsiness and watery vomiting.

YELLOW FEVER

Yellow fever spreads through 'infected' female mosquito called *Aedes aegypti*. The incubation period is 3 to 6 days. Yellow fever countries are western and central Africa and parts of South America. International regulations require proof of yellow fever vaccination for travel to and from these countries. **According to Taber's cyclopedic medical dictionary (1990 edition):** "Except for a few cases in Trinidad in 1954, **urban yellow fever has not been reported in North or South America since 1942.** Outbreaks do occur in Africa adjacent to rain forests. Yellow fever has not been reported in Asia or the eastern coast of Africa". **Then why this mandatory regulation on Yellow Fever?**

Even though the yellow fever infections are mild and can easily be prevented and treated with fruit diet and homeopathy, these mad procedures are followed, like ECT is given routinely to schezophrenics in modern medicine hospitals. Medicine madness, did you say? Indeed it is.

There are two kinds of yellow fever, spread by two different cycles of infection.

Jungle yellow fever is mainly a disease of monkeys. It is spread from infected mosquitoes to monkeys in the tropical rain forest. People get jungle yellow fever when they put themselves in the middle of this natural cycle and are bitten by mosquitoes that have been infected by monkeys. Jungle yellow fever is rare and occurs mainly in persons who work in tropical rain forests.

Urban yellow fever is a disease of humans. It is spread by mosquitoes that have been infected by other people. It is carried from human to human. These mosquitoes have adapted to living among humans in cities, towns, and villages. They breed in discarded tires, flower pots, oil drums, and water storage containers close to human dwellings. Urban yellow fever is the cause of most yellow fever outbreaks and epidemics.

Symptoms: start 3 to 6 days after the bite and can be diagnosed by a blood test. Disease begins with sudden onset of fever, sometimes accompanied by a chill, followed by pain in ear, back and limbs.

Temperature rises rapidly till it reaches 103 to 105°F (39.4 to 40.6°C). Face flushed, conjunctivae injected, pupils small, gastroenteritis, urine scanty and albuminous. This stage lasts from a few hours to several days. It is followed by a marked fall in temperature and an improvement in general symptoms. In the second stage 3 to 9 days, fever rises which can lead to shock, bleeding, and kidney and liver failure. Liver failure causes yellowing of the skin and the whites of the eyes, which gives yellow fever its name. Vomiting is persistent and vomitus may contain dark blood. Due to exhaustion or uremia there may be emergency, but recovery is possible even from gravest condition.

Allopathic Treatment: Dehydration and electrolyte balance will be controlled by IV replacement therapy. Vitamin K and calcium gluconate will be administered for hemorrhagic tendency. *Heparin* will be given in intravascular coagulation. *Dopamine* will be given to maintain blood pressure which does not respond to fluid administration and analgesics for pain. In other words, the Yellow fever has weakened the body, infected liver, kidneys and they will further burden the system.

In Naturopathy, absolute rest in cool, well-ventilated room and liquid diet will be prescribed. The fever will be brought down by plain water enemas, compresses, various baths and by administering fresh fruit juices, coconut water, clear soups, cold herbal teas, lemon-barley water, fresh butter milk (unrefrigerated), mud packs on abdomen and spine, etc. Red Onion Juice and Cayenne Pepper mixed with honey may be applied in the mouth.

Mosquitoes that spread yellow fever usually bite during the day. Travelers should take steps to reduce contact with mosquitoes. When outside: Wear clothes covering the full body. Use insect repellent on exposed skin. When inside: Stay in well-screened areas as much as possible. Use a bednet when sleeping in a room that is not screened or air conditioned. Burn dry Neem leaves or any other safer/herbal mosquito coil to repel the mosquitoes.

Crotalus horridus (potentised Rattlesnake poison)**:-** is the specific homeopathic remedy for Yellow fever. Useful in haemorrhage from any orifice. Passive, dark, unclotted blood in very sick, weakened persons with fever. Headache, worse from jar, must walk on tiptoe. Deathly nausea, vomiting of blood. Chill crawling up and down back, later all over. Yellow colour of the whole body, jaundice. Bruised pain in the bones, with numbness.

Other homeopathic medicines indicated are:
Arsenicum album: as a preventive.

Cadmium sulph: Black discolouration of tongue with yellow fever.

Cantharis: chills running up the back, vomiting of blood streaked membrane and retching, haemorrhages from all orifices.

*Carbo vegetabilis:*Black discolouration of tongue with yellow fever. For the third stage of yellow fever, when there are haemorrhages, with paleness of the face, violent headache, with great heaviness of the limbs and trembling of the body.

Daphne indica: Violent shaking chill, lasting almost twelve hours, followed by heat of moderate duration. Head feels as if skull would burst.

Ipecac: useful in the first stage.

Lachesis mutus - Chill runs up the back, chills with chattering of the teeth, intense left sided throbbing headache, in waves; when there are haemorrhages of blackish non-coagulable blood.

Leptandra virginica: A liver remedy, with jaundice and black, tarry stools. Bilious states. Enfeebled portal circulation. Tongue coated yellow. Aching in region of liver extending to spine, which feels chilly. Weakness, hardly able to stand and walk.

Phosphorus: Yellow fever, haemorrhagic form with petechial spots and small, quick pulse, viscid night sweats. Dry tongue and lips. Vomiting of undigested food soon after eating.

Terebinthina - Ozonised oil of turpentine, a few drops on sugar, several times a day, is recommended as a prophylactic.

TROPICAL FRUITS AND HERBS

God's Pharmacy consists of exotic plants and herbs. But instead of benefiting from them, man looks for artificial medicines and vitamins. That is why he is sick today and looking for heaven after death. A paradise lost.

The value of fruits, flowers, vegetables and herbs to our lives and to our health cannot be over stated. Since our ancestors first walked the earth, they have formed the basis of medicine chests, cosmetic bowls, culinary spice jars, perfume vials and dye pots.

Plants are the source of real food for all life forms. They utilize sunshine, oxygen, water and organic minerals in the process of photosynthesis to feed and grow. They contain glucose, protein, fatty acids, organic minerals, organic enzymes (vitamins) and water (pure). All plants have healing properties as they contain a variety of biologically active substances. The multitude of uses for herbs as foods, medicines and products go to show how vital plants are to our health and well being.

Most herbs in their natural state are safe, and do not leave a residue in the body that could produce side effects. With the use of fruits, vegetables and herbs one could avoid getting sick in the first place because they help to balance and support the body.

Herbs can affect biological systems in our bodies at the cellular and organ level. Ultimately these high levels of biologically active substances can produce pharmacological and therapeutic effects. The nutritional value of herbs is very high and organically grown herbs offer maximum benefits.

In herbal medicine, the various parts of a plant may be used, such as, root, rhizome, stem, leaf, flower, fruit and seed or tissues, bark and wood, or gums and resins. Whole small herbs are used in infusion, or made into tea, others are used as decoction. Other preparations include tinctures, often one part of the herb in five parts of diluted alcohol, or liquid extracts, tablets, pills, lotions, suppositories and inhalants.

There are thousands of herbs and fruits spread all over the world. Listed below are some of the tropical fruits, vegetables and herbs which are useful in the treatment of tropical and other diseases.

Some of the tropical fruits are: Apple, Avocado, Bael Fruit, Banana, Blackberries, Breadfruit, Cashew, Carambola, Coconut, Custard Apple, Durian, Fig, Grapes, Guava, Jackfruit, Jujube, Kiwi, Lemon and Lime, Lychee, Mango, Noni, Oranges, Papaya, Passion Fruit, Peaches, Pineapple, Pomegranate, Rambutan, Rumberry, Sapote, Strawberries, Tamarind, and Water Melon.

Some of the tropical vegetables are: Beetroot, Cabbage, Cauli-flower, Capsicums, Carrots, Cucumber, Green beans, Gourds, Mushrooms, Onions, Peas, Potatoes, Pumpkins, Radish, Sweet potato, Turnips, Tomatoes, Okra, and Leafy vegetables like Amarynth, Fenugreek, Lettuce, Radish and Spinach.

Some of the tropical herbs are: Ashwagandha, Betel Leaf, Cardamom, Clove, Curry Leaves, Drumstick, Ephedra, Garlic, Henna, Kokam, Nutmeg, Pepper, Plumeria, Rainbow Eucalyptus, Sweet Acacia, Winter's Bark, Yerba Mate.

Plants, vegetables, fruits and herbs have within them the healing power, the *Life Force* or *Prana*. Hence, ripe fruits, fresh vegetables, herbs which give immediate relief, sprouts which nourish, soups that revive are recommended during illnesses by Holistic Healers. Hopefully, the so-called qualified doctors will learn this native wisdom and stop playing blind man's bluff game with the patients by prescribing them more and more chemical medicines and insisting that they are life saving. How can anti-biotics (anti-life) be life saving?

DIET IN TROPICAL DISEASES

Real Food is provided by Nature as raw fruits and vegetables. They contain all that is required by the body to be in the healthy state. If food has been processed, cooked or altered in any way so as to change or eliminate any of the natural ingredients, it is not acceptable by the human body.

Any form of processing nature's foods (such as pasteurization, cooking, adding preservatives, etc.) breaks the bonds between the food components and their attached enzymes as well as destroys the enzyme. The result is inorganic or denatured food components and thus inorganic food. The more we process a food, the less nutrient value it retains. This is because living foods are organic foods. Processed foods, to various degrees, are inorganic or 'dead' foods.

The following is the value-wise hierarchy of food

Raw, fresh and whole, consumed immediately – 100%. Dehydrated or dried - loses 2-5% of nutrient value, dried without chemicals or additives. Frozen - loses 5-30% of nutrient value. Steamed - loses 15-60% of nutrient value. Steamed means the green bean is still a bit crispy (if it's limp, it's cooked). Cooked, baked, broiled, boiled, grilled, steamed too long, loses 40-100% of nutrient value, depending on how long it is cooked. Cooked leftovers micro waved - loses 90 - 99% of nutrient value.Commercially canned foods, fried foods and foods with additives not only lose 100% of their nutrient value, but have toxins added to them

We do not 'catch' a disease or illness; we buy it because of our wrong eating. Disease is nothing more than the body responding to the wrong we have done to it. It is the body's attempt at keeping us alive in response to the wrongs we have inflicted on our bodies. Symptoms are indicators that there is an abnormal condition within the body which is producing a state of 'dis-ease'. Diseases/illnesses/symptoms are the body's attempt to restore health and maintain life.

Therefore, Food = Health. If the food we eat is weak, if it lacks vitality, lacks a charge, then the person ingesting that food will be operating from that lower, less energized level. Chinese call this *Chi*, Japanese call it *Qi* and Indians call it *Ojas shakti or Prana shakti*. It is the invisible life-giving nourishment that flows from the environment (internal and external) into the body. It is sometimes difficult to control our external environment but we have complete control over our internal environment through the food we eat.

Three fundamental natural laws: Nutrition (eating), Motion (exercising) and Oxidation (breathing) govern all forms of animal life. Body produces nearly 150 million new blood cells every minute, and all the RBCs in the body completely renew themselves every 90 days. Therefore, tomorrow's blood, bones, glands and muscles depend on what you eat today. As such, whether you will be healthy, weak or sick depends on what you eat. Human nutrition is the most important problem of life.

A balanced or adequate diet is one that supplies all the needs of the body. We should, therefore, learn how, when, why and what to eat and combine and select our food so faithfully that we make proper eating a fixed habit. For as Ayurveda (the science of life) taught centuries ago: "When diet is wrong, medicine is of no use. When diet is correct, medicine is of no need".

Hippocrates said the same when he said, "Let your food be your medicine". In other words, wrong food causes diseases, correct food cures the diseases.

Now let us look at what is correct and what is not correct.

A healthy blood stream should be 70% alkaline and 30% acidic. But due to our wrong eating habits, this ratio is in inverse proportion. Hence diseases are multiplying. Therefore, you would do well to note the following classifications of food items.

Alkali-forming foods: Almonds, apples, apricots, bananas, beets, berries, cabbage, carrots, cauliflower, celery, cherries, cottage cheese, cucumbers, dates, figs, grapes, grapefruit, lemons, lettuce, melons, milk, oranges, papayas, parsley, peaches, pears, pineapples, potatoes, pumpkins, radish, raisins, sprouts, squash, tomatoes, turnips. Four-fifth of your food intake should be from this group.

Acid-forming foods: Barley, beans, cereals, cakes, cheese, corn, chocolates, coffee, eggs, lentils, macaroni, spaghetti, noodles, meats, nuts except almonds, oatmeal, peas, rice, sugar, tea. One-fifth of your food can be from this group.

Laxative foods: Apples, plums, peaches, oranges, pears, grapefruit, pineapples, grapes, figs, prunes, spinach, cauliflower, tomatoes, lettuce, onions, turnips, celery, parsnips, oatmeal, raisins, green peas, cabbage (raw), carrots, string beans, dandelion greens, beet-top greens, buttermilk, whole wheat, bran.

Constipating foods: White bread, pastry, cornstarch, sago, sweet milk, cheese, eggs (boiled), rice, tea, coffee, salt meat, pickled meat, mixed dishes, spiced foods, white crackers.

Laxative foods will keep your bowels running smooth. Constipating food on the other hand will make you run to the doctor.

It is estimated that over 90% of diseases can be attributed directly or indirectly to an unhealthy digestive system. As Dr. Bernard Jensen (pioneering naturopathic physician in the 60's and 70's) says, "It is the bowel that invariably has to be cared for first, before any effective healing can take place".

Toxins from a polluted and congested bowel constantly seep into the bloodstream and lymph systems. They eventually settle into the weakest areas of the body; then various symptoms develop and are given names according to those areas and the degree of cell degeneration. Unfortunately, it is the symptoms resulting from this toxic overload in the bowel that are generally treated rather than the cause.

As Dr. Jensen puts it, "Every tissue is fed by the blood, which is supplied by the bowel. When the bowel is dirty, the blood is dirty and so on to the organs and tissues". Disease can only be permanently overcome when the 'cause' is addressed, rather than merely treating the symptoms.

Parasites mean: a poorly functioning digestive tract with intestines impacted with faecal material. This is the ideal environment for worms and parasites to grow and multiply. There are over 300 varieties that can live in the human body. World-wide, worms outrank cancer as our deadliest enemy. It has been estimated that 150 million people in America alone have intestinal parasite infestation. Over 55 million American children have worms. Parasite infestation is growing rapidly, due to a lack of raw fruits and vegetables in the diet and an increased consumption of cooked and acid-forming foods, red meats, cokes, etc. Once in the intestinal tract, parasites have easy access to other parts of the body where they cause various symptoms and diseases. They can invade the liver, lungs, brain and cause grave complications. "The germ is nothing; the terrain is everything", thus spake Louis Pasteur a little before dying. But the medicine mafia has continued with his plagiarized premise of germs causing disease, because it suits them.

Water, juice fasts or colonics, exercises, massage, mud packs, castor oil treatment, should help remove the parasites by evacuating the filthy intestinal tract. But why eat junk in the first place and allow the problem to grow? As the Great Buddha said, "Every human being is the author of his own health or disease".

Perfect food: The perfect food consists of honey, cream, hot water, oatmeal, lemon juice, grated apple and ground hazel-nuts which contain all the vitamins. Soak ten almonds in water at night. Remove the skin and take them in the morning with one or two tablespoonfuls of honey. This is a potent brain tonic.

While on vacation or traveling, try to live on yogurts and fruits, fruit juices, *kanji, sauerkraut or kimchi.* (For *Kanji* and *Kimchi* see annexures). By all means taste the exotic local food, but avoid meats, junk food, pickles and refrigerated / recycled food. Instead of popping artificial vitamins, eat tropical fruits rich in vitamins. For example, *Vitamins A, B1, B3, B5, B6, B9, C and E, as also Calcium and Iron,* are found aplenty in tropical fruits and vegetables (see list in chapter titled God's Pharmacy). *Vitamin B12* is found in Fish, Poultry, Meat or dairy products. *Vitamin D* is available in Sunlight, eggyolk, milk, ghee, codliver and salmon liver oil.

HOMEOPATHIC AND BIOCHEMIC MEDICINE IN TROPICAL DISEASES

Even though homeopathic remedies have been outlined in every disease chapter, this chapter will explain the principles of homeopathic and biochemic remedies. I have also discussed homeopathic vaccinations which are safer, cheaper and without side effects.

The idea prevalent in the minds of the general public is that infectious diseases can be cured only by modern medicine. This idea is fallacious. Other systems of medicine have much to offer.

Homeopathy, for example, has been curing these cases ever since **Dr. Samuel Hahnemann** founded the Homeopathic system of medicine in Germany in 1790. The Homeopathic principle, being founded on truth, is as valid today as it was then, and continues to cure people suffering from a wide range of acute and chronic diseases. Homeopathy offers medicines which are gentle, safe and quick in action, provided they have been selected well and the dose adjusted correctly.

Homeopathy does not treat diseases by name. Diseases are often varied in their symptoms during the inception, invasion and course, and often spend their force in different locations of the body, depending on the individual susceptibilities of the patient. Hence, the Homeopathic remedy is selected depending on the symptom picture that a suffering individual displays at that given point in time. It requires detailed observation on the part of both, patient and doctor, to be able to choose the ideal remedy for the patient.

Though remedies have been named in this book according to the disease, it must be borne in mind that these remedies have been selected only because past records show that they have a similar disease picture, and hence have been used often for such conditions. You may consult a Homeopath for proper analysis and treatment. In case patients do choose and take remedies on their own initiative, it is advisable not to continue the same remedy in frequent repetitions over a long period of time. A well-selected remedy works very fast and hence should not be continued for long.

Homeopathic medicines are not drugs in the strict sense; they are remedies. The difference between drugs and remedies is: drugs are coarse, can damage the organs and kill a person, they being toxic. Remedies (like homeopathic, biochemic, flower remedies) are the released energy of the drugs, which help trigger the inbuilt immunity of the body and readjust the equilibrium.

Please always remember that
(a) healing is within;
(b) patient is impatient;
(c) treatment should not be worse than the disease;
(d) it should be affordable;
(e) there is unity of disease and consequently
(f) the unity of healing.

Homeopathy considers the whole personality of the patient, his body, mind and soul, total constitution, personality types, whether the disease is at causal or astral (dynamic) level, and by safety yardstick, homeopathy is the safest.

The cardinal laws of homeopathy are:
(a) the law of similars
(b) the law of drug proving
(c) the principle of potentisation
(d) the theory of chronic diseases
(e) the law of direction of cure
(f) the law of single remedy and
(g) the law of minimum dose and minimum repetition.

Homeopathic remedies are cheaper to buy, lighter to carry on a journey, easy to administer, and the results are immediate, if the remedy is well-selected. These remedies are available in the form of globules or potentised tinctures. **Mother tinctures** (like rescue remedy, crataegus or cactus Q) are not potentised, but are the original dilutions in pure alcohol. These are used in drops, 10 drops to 1 ounce of water; 1 teaspoon = 1 dose. Always use 30 or 200 potencies. Higher potencies like 1M, 10M are used where the condition is severe, or in emergencies. As regard repetition of doses, usually 3 to 4 times a day should suffice in most cases. Then doses are to be reduced to 1 to 2 times (at longer intervals of 12 to 24 hours).

Some Homeo Remedies and their application are given below. Remember these are polycrests, meaning, one remedy can be used in several diseases. Also note that homeopathy works very fast if proper medicine, proper potency, proper time, and proper frequency is used.

Aconite: sudden shock, initial heart attack, great fear and anxiety, swollen tongue, swollen and hard testicles, menses profuse, nightmares.

Arnica: for any injury, external or internal, bruises, wounds, shock due to injury, angina pectoris, fatty heart, weak and falling neck.

Arsenic alb: acute cold, food poisoning, asthma, ascites and dropsy, Bright's disease, diabetic gangrene, flu.

Belladonna: sunstroke, sun headaches, all inflammations, appendicitis and meningitis.

Bryonia: migraine, vertigo, nose bleed, biliousness.

Calendula: antiseptic properties, quick healing in cuts and bruises. In paralysis and as an intercurrent remedy in cancer.

Cantharis: burns and blisters, furious delirium, bladder irritation, pleurisy.

Carbo veg: collapse, shock, air hunger, cold and clammy hands. It can hold a person from dying. Disorders arising from flatulence, which includes even heart attacks.

Dulcamara: paralysis, warts on hands, wet weather diarrhoea, stiff neck.

72

Euphrasia/Cineraria succus maritima eyedrops: Great eye remedies. Euphrasia for conjunctivitis, pressure in eyes, little blisters on cornea. *Cineraria* for cataract.

Hepar sulph: tonsilitis, sore throat, all suppurations, fevers due to, discharge of uterine blood, gonorrhoea.

Kali phos: disorders arising in nervous tissues, for weak eyesight, good for memory, sound sleep, cerebral anaemia, offensive breath.

Ledum: puncture injuries, for snake and spider bites, aching in eyes, gouty pains, anal fissures and piles pain.

Lycopodium: for lichen, liver, and erectile dysfunction. Also for dry and tight vagina.

Mag phos: anti-spasmodic, goitre, muscular and intestinal cramps, neuralgic pains, ptosis.

Merc sol / Plantago: toothache, swollen glands, fever with cold, spongy and bleeding gums, cavities.

Nat mur: for scorpion bite, goitre and diabetes.

Nux vomica: abdominal colic, constipation, jaundice, drug addiction and stress. It is 'the remedy' for modern lifestyles.

Phosphorous: expistaxis, loss of vision, diplopia, acute hepatitis, bleeding piles, AIDS.

Pulsatilla: acute earaches, diarrhoea due to fatty food, ripened cold, hypersensitive and most gynaecological problems; school girls' remedy.

Rhus tox: specific for influenza/SARS, rheumatic pains, bodyaches and over exertion, strain and sprain.

Ruta G: pain from back down hips and buttocks, cramps, sciatica, contraction of fingers. Glioblastoma multiforme (multiple tumours in brain).

Sulphur: eczema, piles, lichen planus and for all skin remedies.

Symphytum with Calc phos for fractures and bones problems like osteoporosis and over calcification.

IMMUNISATION: **Like in other diseases, homoeopathy has clearly established its superiority in treating viral diseases. These medicines (called nosodes) are produced from the diseased products themselves.**

Allopathic immunisation procedure itself is a health hazard. Vaccines wiped out small-pox, polio, diphtheria, typhoid, influenza, we are told. In effect, however, the blood contamination from the vaccines not only causes the same disease in severe and even fatal forms, but the vaccine poisons cause other diseases, such as, paralysis, blindness, brain damage, cancers, autism, etc. **Hence, go in for safer, cheaper and reliable Homeopathic prophylactics, nosodes or vaccines, as under:**

AIDS: Medorrhinum, Syphilinum, Tuberculinum or Thuja. (Also, Echinacea, Lachesis, Sulphur, Phosphorus and Lycopodium).
Cancer: Carcinosin.
Chicken Pox: Malandrinum or Variolinum.
Diphtheria: Diphtherinum or Mercurious Cyanatus.
Gonorrhoea: Medorrhinum.
Infective Hepatitis: Nux Vomica.
Influenza: Arsenic Album.
Measles (Rubella): Morbillinum or Pulsatilla.
Mumps: Morbillinum or Parotidinum.
Polio: Lathyrus or polio nosode.
Rabies: Hydrophobinum (Lyssin).
Syphilis: Syphilinum.
Small Pox: Variolinum.
Tuberculosis: Bacillinum or Tuberculinum.
Typhoid: Ars Alb. or Baptisia.
Whooping Cough: Drosera or Pertussin.

For the after effects of Allopathic Vaccination or Vaccinosis, or to neutralize lethal drugs like AZT - which inhibit bone-marrow production, which in turn necessitates continual blood transfusion for many patients - give Thuja and Kali Mur and lots of fresh curds (yogurts).

Then there are 12 Tissue Salts. These are also known as Schuessler salts after Dr.W.H. Schuessler, MD (1873) of Germany, who called them natural or physiological function remedies. The twelve inorganic (mineral) salts are essential to the proper growth and development of every part of the system.

Given in potentised or trituration forms, these Tissue Salts are quickly assimilated by the body and also help in absorbing natural salts from the food eaten. The 12 Tissue Salts are:

Calcarea fluor (flouride of Lime): promotes elasticity of tissues. Used for piles, ruptures, strained tendons, varicose veins, muscles weakness, stretch marks, circulation problem, cracked tongue and lips.

Calcarea phos (phosphate of Lime): helps build new blood cells, strengthens bones and teeth, aids digestion; used for poor circulation, chilblains, lowered vitality, muscle weakness, iron deficiency anaemia, decaying teeth and teething problems.

Calcarea sulph (sulphate of Lime): a blood constituent and purifier, for spots during adolescence, slow healing skin and wounds, sore lips.

Ferrum phos (phosphate of Iron): constituent of red blood cells which helps to distribute oxygen in the body; used for inflammation in general, feverishness, chestiness, sore throat, coughs, colds, chills, and muscular rheumatism.

Kali mur (chloride of Potash): asthma and bronchitis, colds, tonsillitis, sluggish digestion.

Kali phos (phosphate of Potash): a nerve soother and nutrient, used for tension, headaches, depression, loss of sleep, irritability due to worry and excitement and indigestion.

Kali sulph (sulphate of Potash): promotes and maintains healthy skin. For discharge from the nose and throat, poor condition of nails, hair and scalp.

Magnesium phos (phosphate of Magnesia): nerve and muscle fibre nutrient. Used to relieve darting pains, cramps and menstrual pain, acute spasms, hiccups, colic and wind.

Natrum mur (chloride of Soda): controls distribution of water in the body. Used for watery colds with flow of tears and runny nose; loss of smell or taste.

Natrum phos (phosphate of Soda): acid-alkaline regulator of the cells. Used for acidity, heart burns, gastric indigestion and rheumatic pains.

Natrum sulph (sulphate of Soda): balances body water, used for queasiness, morning sickness, digestive problems, bilious attacks, colic, influenza and headaches.

Silicea (Silica): conditioner and cleanser, eliminates waste. Used for toxic accumulation, pimples and spots, boils, styes.

Before we end this chapter, an introduction to **Genus Epidemicus** or remedies useful in particular region and epidemic, would be useful.

During each epidemic, a competent local Homeopath closely studies symptoms common to the majority of the people afflicted during that period and place, and thus gets the total picture of the specific epidemic. He then matches the 'picture' called 'symptom totality' of that epidemic with the homeopathic 'remedy picture' or pictures of a relevant remedy or remedies available in his Materia Medica. There must be one or two remedies whose 'symptom totality' closely resembles or matches with the presenting totality of epidemic syndrome then raging. These selected remedies are called *Genus Epidemicus,* since they are relevant to the type of epidemic and are spefically curative in every case, as well as act as preventive.

My conclusion based on 35 years as Holistic Physician: Allopathy multiplies diseases, cons, controls, maims and kills patients. Homeopathy cures diseases and restores patients back to health. But Diet is the ultimate in curing diseases and restoring health. Hence, adopt Diet with Detox, Biochemic or Homeopathic remedies and Yoga as the ultimate in Holistic Healing.

ANTHROPOSOPHIC MEDICINE
Dilnawaz Bana and Kashmira Rebello

In this chapter, to round up the discussion on Holistic Healing Arts, we introduce you to Anthroposophic Medicine (AM in short).

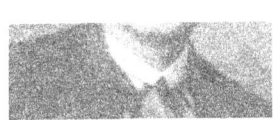

In 1921, the Austrian philosopher **Dr. Rudolf Steiner** (1861-1925) was approached by European physicians to formulate guidelines for the application of Anthroposophy, which Steiner had developed, to the field of standard medicine. Steiner presented a series of 21 discourses on "Spiritual Science and Medicine" at the Goetheanum, at Dornach, Switzerland. He taught European doctors to look at the Human Being in relation to health and illness, according to the higher cosmic laws, which sustain life on earth. Thus was born Anthroposophic Medicine.

One of the attending physicians was Dr. Ita Wegman (1876-1943) with whom Steiner collaborated in writing *Fundamentals of Therapy: An extension of the Art of Healing through Spiritual Knowledge,* in 1925. Shortly thereafter, Wegman founded a medical clinic at Arlesheim, near Basel, Switzerland, for the practice of AM and she also began producing its distinctive pharmacopoeia.

Steiner's views are holistic in nature and "Goethean" in approach. Each part of the human being is related to the whole and the whole represented in every part of the organism. The forces of metamorphosis activate the organism and give each individual the uniqueness of personality. Every event in the life of a person is also a part in the wholeness of one's destiny and connected most intrinsically and intimately with the organism.

There are four essential aspects to the human being – physical body, life body, soul body and ego organization. Human potential goes far beyond the capacities of the mechanical model. The true measure of man is a universal measure belonging to the whole of creation, where man has the whole of the natural world in him, and nature is an infinitely differentiated human being, as Paracelsus put it.

77

Man has the whole of the natural world in him; nature is an infinitely differentiated human being.

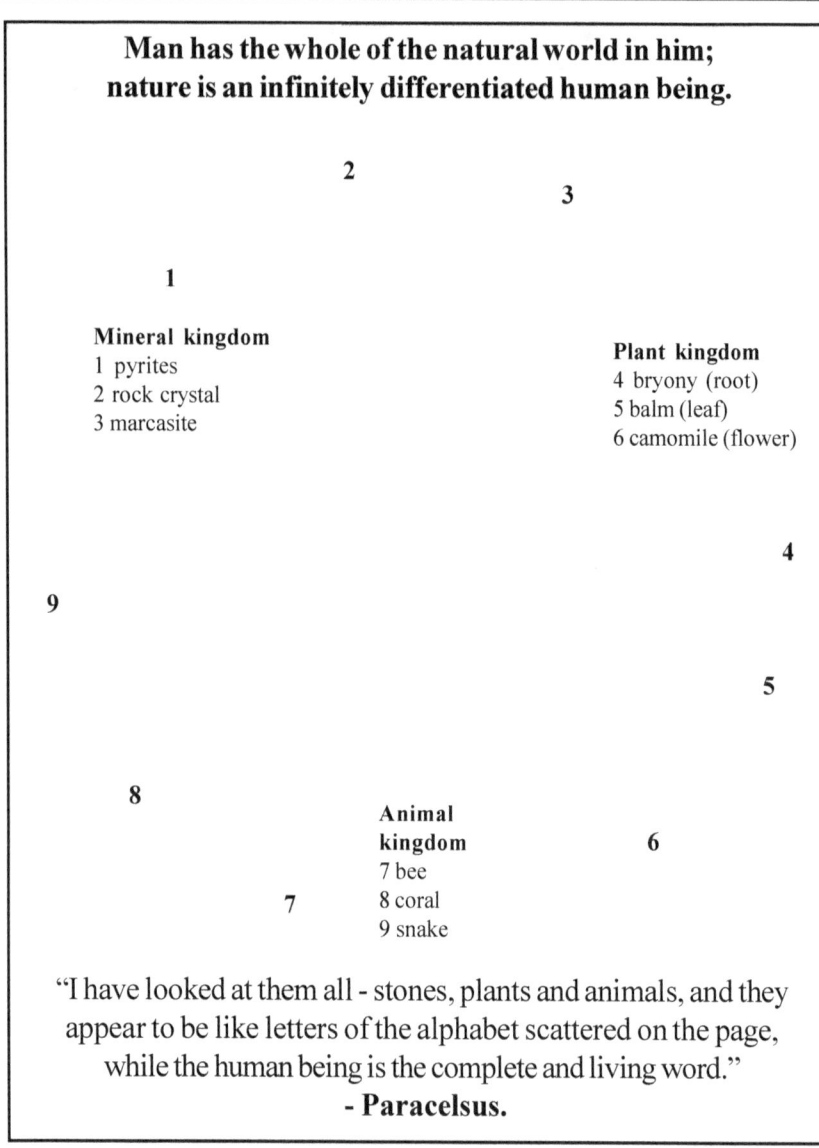

2

3

1

Mineral kingdom
1 pyrites
2 rock crystal
3 marcasite

Plant kingdom
4 bryony (root)
5 balm (leaf)
6 camomile (flower)

4

9

5

8

Animal kingdom
7 bee
8 coral
9 snake

6

7

"I have looked at them all - stones, plants and animals, and they appear to be like letters of the alphabet scattered on the page, while the human being is the complete and living word."
- Paracelsus.

So, in nature as also in humans, one sidedness means getting separated from the whole, like falling out of paradise. With the fall come illnesses as tipping over of a balance. Thus, restoring balance, making whole or healing, happens on a higher level, on a new consciousness. The effort to overcome illness brings a sense of inner freedom. In a higher sense, every illness or suffering is a stage of development for the human being. Many people actually feel renewed after an illness. Through this experience they metamorphose into totally different humans. This 'insight gained in illness' offers knowledge of becoming healthy, rather than remain placid. It is a process which assimilates a new dimension in one's personality.

Unfortunately, chemically based, hard-drug oriented medicine can rob the person of precious freedom to receive nature-oriented treatment which all organisms deserve. This is where AM steps in and permits the person to re-establish health. The whole point is to enable the patient to find 'own healing'.

Since time immemorial, the 'trinity based approach' has been implemented in a number of traditional forms of medicine. Be it Ayurveda, which talks of *Kafa* (phlegm), *Pita* (bile) and *Vata* (gas), or the Paracelsian trinity of Salt, Mercury and Sulphur, humanity has experienced the threefold based treatment on all levels, from the physical to the spiritual. The Anthroposophical approach too distinguishes three systems:

1. The *sensory-nervous system,* which is primarily located in the head, relates to thinking.

2. The *rhythmical system,* primarily located in the region of the chest, relates to feeling.

3. The *metabolic-limb system,* which is located in the limbs and digestive organs, relates to the will or the action aspect of our personality

This threefold system is not only interconnected, but is constantly interacting in a healthy person. The polar opposite systems are a landscape of the person; winter, relating to the head pole of the sensory-nervous system and summer, relating to the limb pole of the digestive-metabolic system. Both these systems should communicate with each other in the rhythmical system of the heart region. Here the balance is maintained.

These two systems are not only polar opposites, like the summer and winter poles of the earth, but one system creates, the other destroys. The spring and autumn part of nature could be likened to the rhythmical system, which in turn intermediates between warmth and coolness, harmonizing the destructive effects of the one and the creative effects of the other. Here lies the strength of metabolism, anabolism and catabolism.

Both the warmth and the cooling systems are of utmost importance to regulate the bodily temperature. In case the warm pole of the metabolic system overlaps or dominates or suppresses the cool pole of the sensory-nervous system or *vice versa*, then the entire system is thrown off balance. This may lead either to inflammatory or to hardening illnesses and problems, not only of the body but of the mind as well. For instance, migraine is warmth on the wrong side of the body.

With the threefold nature of the person, Steiner brings into awareness a fourfold principle, relating to the four main elements of earth, water, air and fire, with their respective temperaments and constitutions.

1. The physical body, with earth as its element, relates to the mineral kingdom.

2. The etheric or life body, with water as its element, relates to the plant kingdom.

3. The astral body, with air as its element, relates to the animal kingdom.

4. The Ego organization or the consciousness of the Self, with fire as its element, relates to the Spirit in the Human Being.

These four systems intermingle with each other, one dominating the other to create innumerable variations, physically, emotionally and mentally.

The holistic methods of supporting the patient's health-giving forces are not only through diversely prepared AM, but also through healing movements of Eurythmy. Included are also baths, massage and relevant art therapies like painting, sculpture, speech formation and music therapy. All these combined with proper nourishment and therapeutic lifestyles of moderation signify a complete sense of the term 'holistic'.

Where conventional medicine concentrates solely on destroying the agents of disease, suppressing associated processes and replacing missing substances (e.g. vitamins, hormones, blood elements), AM aims to enable the human organism to overcome a disease through its own resources (patient's powers of self-healing). The emphasis is on restoring the balance of bodily functions and strengthening the immune system. The right medicines play a major role in this process.

AM uses mineral, vegetable, metal, and animal-based raw materials in the production of medicines. For instance, quartz, sulphur, and lime are typical mineral substances, while arnica, yellow gentian, and chamomile are well-known medicinal herbs. Of the metals, gold, silver, iron and tin are frequently used, while animal-based substances include insect venom.

Steiner indicated subtle cosmic connections among the 7 principal metals (silver, lead, mercury, tin, copper, iron, and gold), the stars, planets, Sun, Moon, and the major body organs. For example, Mars/iron/gall bladder and Venus/copper/kidney are recognized correspondences. Steiner also developed Bidor, made from silica, iron and sulphur. Bidor works in establishing harmony in the body and is used to treat migraine, which occurs when the system goes whack. Silica, which relates to the nerve-sense pole, selflessly lets the light in, like eyes; sulphur relates to the warmth process of the metabolic-limb system; and iron mediates between both poles in the blood, in the rhythmic system. Among herbs, *Equisetum,* in its essential nature is correlated with the kidney, *primula* for the heart, *dandelion* for the liver, *bryophyllum* for the lungs.

Another medicinal category suggested by Steiner is "compositions on the model of curative plants", for example, *solutio siliceae, solutio alkalina and solutio ferri.* "Type remedies" are modeled after the basic processes in the human or specific organs in their archetypal functioning. They represent the equalizing of certain antagonisms between selected plants and minerals. There are many examples of type remedies, such as, *cardiodoron, hepatodoron, choleodoron, combudoron, digestodoron, menodoron* – all formulated and named by Steiner. He had the notion of *doron* as 'gift of'. Thus, *cardiodoron* is 'gift of the heart'; made principally with primrose, a type remedy that embraces the totality of the functions of the heart and circulation.

Hepatodoron, which activates the archetypal nature of the liver function, is made from leaves of the wild strawberry and grapvine. *Choleodoron,* for the treatment of gall bladder dysfunctions, is made of celandine and turmeric and has been used successfully by Dr. Victor Bott in over 500 cases of gall stones, obviating surgery. *Digestodoron,* made from varieties of willow and fern, is used to treat rhythmic disturbances of the gastrointestinal tract, while *Menodoron,* made from oak bark, marjoram seed, nettles, and yarrow, is effective for menstrual disorders.

The patient can be treated by various different routes: by means of the senses, the digestive system, the respiratory system and the bloodstream. What response the doctor is seeking to stimulate in the body determines the form of access taken. Compresses, rubs, or packs using tinctures, ointments, or essential oils, for instance, stimulate the nervous system via the skin and the senses. This encourages forming and structuring processes to take place.

Drops, globuli, syrups and powders influence the digestive system and stimulate regenerative, dynamic processes. When inhaled or injected, substances enter the body's circulation directly and have an immediately balancing effect. The means by which a medicine is administered is therefore of considerable importance, since the body reacts differently to the various methods. When applied externally as oil, *lovage (levisticum),* for instance, has an anti-inflammatory effect on neuritis and otitis media acuta; when taken internally as drops, it stimulates the digestion.

Some anthroposophic medicines contain poisons, e.g. deadly nightshade (belladonna), foxglove (digitalis), monkshood (aconitum), and strychnine (Strychnos nux-vomica). However, as with all medicines, following the correct dosage ensures safety in use. Moreover, such medicines are only prescribed in small packs, so that even if the patient were to take the medication incorrectly (i.e. ingest the contents of an entire pack), no serious or incurable symptoms of poisoning would arise.

Anthroposophic medicines are now available worldwide. Here are some and their indications:

Arnica/Betula Comp. (50 ml) for cerebral arteriosclerosis, hypertension.

Arsenicosum D-15 (50 ml) an acute remedy for Asthma.

Cactus/Magnesia Phos D6 (50 ml) in acute attack of ischaemic heart disease.

Capsella Bursa Pastoris D4 (20 ml): an anti-haemorrhagic and anti uric acid remedy; uterine haemorrhage with cramps and expulsion of clots; albuminuria during gestation; chronic cystitis; dysuria and spasmodic retention; chronic neuralgia; haemorrhage from uterine fibroid with back ache or renal and vesical irritation.

Pancreas D6 (20 ml): principal action on pancreas; pancreatic dysfunction; pancreatitis.

Passiflora Inc. D4 (20 ml) for insomnia; worm fever, teething, spasms.

Sabal Serrulata D1 (20 ml) in prostate enlargement; epididymitis and urinary difficulties; valuable for undeveloped mammary glands.

Amara trophen (50 ml): reflux oesophagitis.

Avena Sativa Comp. (50 ml) nerve tonic, anxiety, sleeplessness.

Berberis, planta tota/Urtica urens (50 gms) for uterine fibroids.

Melissa Cupro culta, ren D3 (50 ml) for harmonizing renal and urogenital functions.

Ovarium D3 (20 ml) for ovarian cyst, harmonizing ovarian functions.

The root cause of any disease is imbalance in the system. Environmental factors may aggravate to an extent, but they are not responsible for a disease.

During travel, for example, apart from jetlag, one may have injuries or illnesses due to indiscretions, all which have been described in detail in this book.

REMEDIAL EURYTHMY
By Dilnawaz Bana

Eurythmy is a movement linked to the sounds of speech. Certain movements represent the vowel sounds, others the consonants. It is used for many physical and mental disorders. It is also very beneficial for children, developing their suppleness and sense of rhythm.

In 1912 Dr. Rudolf Steiner brought a new art of movement into existence on the foundation of Anthroposophy. "Anthropos" in Greek means the human being, striving through the inner wisdom or consciousness, "Sophia" – to receive the outer wisdom or consciousness of the universe.

Dr. Steiner talks of Anthroposophy as having its roots in the perceptions already gained in the spiritual world. The branches, leaves, blossoms and fruits of Anthroposophy grow into all the fields of human life and action.

Anthroposophy has brought new light of consciousness into every field of life, from creative education, arts and science to medicine, architecture, social sciences, bio-dynamic farming and a new art of movement called Eurythmy (rythmy is written without an "h", being a Greek word).

This new art is not a dance, nor a mime but an art of movement, making visible the "Eu"-beauty and harmony of sound in speech and music and creating a new health-giving rhythm in the organism. Thus, Eurythmy is speech and music made visible through conscious movement of the limbs.

Eurythmy uses for its expression the most flexible of all instruments, the human body. It knows no limitations in its possibility for the development of body, mind and soul.

One can perceive the human organism as microcosmos, mirroring or containing the macrocosmos. As Paracelsus (1494-1541), a Swiss mystic and doctor says: "The human being is a spread out macrocosmos and the macrocosmos is a condensed human being." Each part and particle in nature is a sound and the human being – the WORD!

Sounds contain wisdom, laws and mystery of the universe. Sounds made visible through conscious movement of the limbs in Eurythmy, make these very laws more real and unlock step by step the dynamic force behind the tangible world.

These are the very forces, which are working in us, sustaining our organism. The formative forces of the cosmos create the very fabric of our being. The whole universe is created out of sound with its seed in OM or AUM.

Every organ, every breath we take and even a single thought is in relationship to the dynamic forces around us. Our roots are in the universe, mirroring the undying spirit behind our individuality, giving us the power to strive over and above our physical boundaries.

With this in mind, every sound made visible, works therapeutically. Each sound is in tune with the health giving formative forces working in our organs, in our organism, in our very breathing.

Invoking these sounds, activating them through the movements of Eurythmy, we strengthen a general feeling of wellbeing. Not only that but Eurythmy is differentiated, since each sound is also differentiated in its structure, and the process of its unfolding is highly curative for any particular illness, be it of the psychosomatic kind, chronic or acute.

At the same time, when one experiences the sound through the movement with full attention, one is striving step by step to unlock the mystery, the beauty and the wisdom of the universe. Yet the most difficult of all instruments of the world – the human body – is not so easy to play in tune and in harmony with the world around us. That is why the average human being is not able to hold the full impact of this dynamic force, all at once. This way, our guardian of the Threshold protects us, since any shortcut may prove to be harmful. It is a step by step process to lift the veil of Isis, the Reality behind the veil of *maya*.

This Reality is the very fabric of our organism. When the sound is made visible one comes nearer to the essence, which lies behind the existence. Rudolf Steiner has developed Eurythmy along a threefold aspect. First, as a performing art; secondly pedagogical, as group Eurythmy for children and adults; and thirdly, therapeutically as curative Eurythmy. They have now been adopted in Rudolf-Steiner-Clinics, hospitals, institutions and homes.

Dr. Steiner has given innumerable indications for curative Eurythmy for various physical and mental problems. These curative exercises are to be done under the anthroposophical doctor's guidance with a curative Eurythmist, otherwise the same may be harmful.

This is the first time these exercises are given in a book-form and for this reason, I have, in collaboration with Dr. Leo Rebello, simplified them so that these exercises work more for the General Wellbeing of the individual without having to go into details of treating a specific disorder.

I have worked as a curative Eurythmist since 1977 in different hospitals and clinics of Germany and Switzerland. My years of experience has taught me that curative Eurythmy is a Process. It works on a very subtle level and its in-depth therapeutic activity is a long-lasting transformation of the body, mind and soul. As a patient, one is an alchemist, transforming the gross into the subtle, the heaviness of lead into gold. This process has its own time – chronos – for the overall wellbeing of the organism because the effort one puts in is the most important aspect.

Through Eurythmy one experiences health in its totality, since the path of working consciously for health is a path of knowledge.

The three soul functions of thinking, feeling and willing, represented by the central nervous system, the rhythmical system and the metabolic digestive system, overcome the darkness of one-sidedness, bringing these three main systems into one whole. Thus, health means "making whole".

Curative Eurythmy exercises are represented by sequences of sounds, combining vowels or consonants or both, each sound representing each movement of the limbs. One repeats the movements, bringing full attention to what one is doing, with open eyes and breathing according to one's own normal rhythm. Never stress, hold or strain the breath, nor any particular thought, but bring your full attention to whatever movement you are practicing.

These indications of therapeutic movements in this book, comprising vowels and consonants, are remedial, preventive and prophylactic.

Normally, practicing under the guidance of an Anthroposophical doctor and a curative Eurythmist, the sound sequence takes on the role of "medicinal movements", each session lasting a half to one full hour, done three to five times a week. Later on, the patient discharged from the clinic, tries out the prescribed exercises at home for several weeks or even months.

Complete study to become a curative Eurythmist can extend up to six years with the basics of sound-study, which also includes subjects like speech formation, painting, sculpturing, geometry and basic study of anatomy and physiology with its dynamic functioning in the organism. I would be sidestepping if I were to describe the study of the dynamic functioning as well, because that includes the subtle members of the physical body like the etheric body, the astral body and the higher Ego.

In curative Eurythmy the movements of the sounds made visible, imitate the healthy functioning not only of the organism but of each specific organ as well.

When one learns Eurythmy sequences of sound and movement through a book, one has to observe certain precautions. First and foremost, these exercises are meant for people over 16 years of age. It is risky for children under 16, though curative Eurythmy may be given to them under expert advice. Another important point to note is, that curative Eurythmy is not a miracle cure.

Though one can strengthen one's immune system and mobilise the "inner doctor", the outer doctor should not be ignored. It is to bring one's attention only on the movement one is doing, breathing normally. Do not close your eyes unnecessarily, nor try to breathe according to the eurythmical movement. Also do not utter the sound because when you move the sound, you are the sound. So please keep your mouth closed whilst doing Eurythmy. Thereby, the whole organism is thinking, feeling and willing at the same time. No music is required for any extra support, lest one's attention gets divided. Wait at least an hour after meals; otherwise no definite time is imposed. Be free to chart out your own time when you do your exercises. Also, the length of the exercise should be kept free. Do not "overdose".

About 10 to 20 minutes, three to five times a week, continue to practice for six to seven weeks. Thereafter, take a break from the exercises for one and a half to two weeks. You may start again, if you wish with the same exercises. Do all these exercises slowly.

Since Dr.Rebello details the holistic healing in tropical illnesses, my area is to describe in a nutshell, the Eurythmy movements.

The first and most important exercise to start and end a session of Eurythmy is the jewel called the IAO. Three movements are given on three basic vowels. EE as in eat, AA as in ask, and O as in open. Please note that the movements correspond to the sound and not the written letter.

Stand consciously, quietly with your eyes open and free gaze. Do not stare at anything. Put your feet together.

Now relax your back (not too deep), your arms and knees (Fig 1). Then slowly lift yourself up in an upright position without straining yourself (Fig 2).

1   Feel your spine, arms and shoulders are relaxed   2
without any undue pressure in any area. Feel yourself
connected upwards and downwards.

In this position of the sound EE feel yourself as a personality, radiant and full of Inner Light of your consciousness. Feel the space on which you stand with feet firmly on the ground and your head as if touching the dome of the sky. This feeling of your entire personality – I am I – is in response to the inner mood of the light-filled sound of EE.

Maintain this upright position and now take a step sideways with one leg and then the other leg, without losing the centre of the space on which you stand. With feet astride, anchor yourself firmly on the ground (Fig 3). This position of standing earthbound with open legs corresponds to the open sound of AA. Now without losing these two positions, the vertical linear EE and the open AA, proceed towards the third sound O.   3

Here we form a circle at the chest level (Fig 4), the fingertips lightly touching each other. The arms are held without any tension. Shoulders are relaxed. The arms are now creating an inner space as if enclosing a sphere of light. Hold all three positions consciously for a moment and then one by one, release all three, first releasing the arms (the O) then release the AA by bringing the feet together again and then release the EE, which means relax a bit as in Fig 1. Immediately repeat the entire procedure, building the EE once more, then the AA and then the O, release one by one all the three positions to build them over and over again at least five to seven times. Release and build, release and build.

4

Now this exercise forms a unity of our threefold system. The head and spine with its central nervous system, the lower limbs corresponding to the metabolic digestive system and the heart sphere with the arms, corresponding to the rhythmical system.

These three systems also represent the soul forces of thinking, willing and feeling, respectively. EE, AA, O is beneficial and remedial for all one-sided problems like having a warm head and cool limbs instead of the other way around. This brings a balance between the polarity of the head and the limb system, forming a centre through the rhythmical system. Therefore, EE, AA and O should accompany the start and the end of all subsequent exercises.

Every sound, which holds in itself the laws of the universe, has also innumerable descriptions. One has to experience their subtle working by repeating the corresponding movements of the sounds. One has the freedom to make one's own observations through proper practice. The three sound exercise for Jaundice or viral Hepatitis B – LMO.

Since Dr. Rebello has already described the illness I will describe the movements based on the three corresponding sounds of LMO.

L is a fluid sound, having water as its element. L releases bodily congestion, working on the formative principle of directional flow of fluids in the body. Let us now try out the movement of L.

Sit or stand with your spine comfortably erect. Try to visualise how rainwater collects into the earth, rises, condenses and falls into the earth again. You may picture the sap, which through the roots, rises in the bark of the tree and frees itself upwards in the light of the sun, as branches, leaves, flowers and fruits completing the cycle, going downwards and gathering itself again into the earth.

As nature circulates the wheel of life, similarly one circulates the movements. Start from the downward movement, dipping the arms from both the sides as if collecting precious liquid (Fig 5). Bring the arms together and then raise the

5

6   7   8

arms (Fig 6) upwards until the level of the head (Fig 7) and then allow the arms to separate sideways opening the fingers (Fig 8) 9 bringing the arms slowly start 10 start downwards (Fig 9), continue the cycle about five to seven times. It is a circular movement. Slowly, deliberately, the L movement imitates the whole cycle of the rising and falling of the water. It looks like this, when complete (Fig 10).

As mentioned, visualise the pattern of the movement with full attention. After this refreshing L done a few times in continuity, transfer your attention to the Sound M with its corresponding movement. M is a resonance sound and if the resonance is transferred to the movement of the arms, then it is a give-and- take, out-and-in, to-and-fro movement.

Now, if the give-and-take of our daily existence, like out-and-in breathing is imitated, with the movement of the arms, then there is an exchange of warmth. This warmth is only possible if held in balance.

Thus M helps to create equilibrium within the bodily warmth. It is truly an exchange of warmth, not only on the bodily level but also on the social level: It's a constant striving, constant struggle to keep one's destiny in balance, between too much or too little.

12

14

11

13

After the L sound-movement, start the M by bringing your hands onto the chest level, palms facing outwards (Fig 11). Visualize or imagine that you are slowly feeling through something dense, slowly reaching out to touch, to feel the outside world with your fingertips, extending your arms outwards. (Fig 12) Do not overstretch your arms.

Now turn your extended arms inwards, palms facing you and slowly bring your hands towards you as if you are bringing something precious, all the time remaining at the chest level (Fig 13).

Repeat the M three to four times and then transfer your attention to the sound O and its corresponding round movement, enclosing space at the chest level. Make this movement only once.

Repeat the whole exercise LMO two to three times, first the L a few times, M a few times and O only once. LMO nourishes, refreshes and creates a healthy new rhythm in the body, also working against depressive outlook on life. LMO imitates the healthy functioning of the entire metabolic system, especially the liver, releasing congestion to purify the system, regulating warmth and creating a proper boundary, so that the toxins do not infiltrate the surrounding organs.

Finish off the LMO by one vigorous crossing of the arms, sound movement A (as in ate) at chest level (Figure 14). Feel the point of crossing for sometime and release. A, will give further strength to LMO.

Let us now advance to the two other major problems, which are prevalent in the tropics: Malaria and Dengue both caused by the mosquito.

We will take into account both these illnesses with a highly remedial exercise, the threefold walking and then with one supporting vowel, AA (as in ask).

The first major exercise is called the threefold walking. This is a very helpful exercise to focus our thinking, feeling and willing in one single unity. The very name Malaria means bad (mal) air (aria). We will have to try and purify the "bad air" in us, overcoming this particular susceptibility, which made us a prey in the first place to the bite of the mosquito. The following exercise harmonises the entire system. Start with the IAO and then do the slow and steady threefold walk.

For this walk, one needs only walking space – small or large does not make much of a difference because the goal lies within each part of a step. In this exercise there is nothing like reaching a particular place.

In the threefold walking, each step consists of three parts. First, stand normally, spine upright and no undue tension. Imagine that you are wearing a precious crown of gold, which lightens up your head. If you move your head up or down or sideways the crown falls and you would have to wear it again. So keep your head steady. Feet are firmly feeling the ground. Stand at the end of the room but do not fix your gaze, nor is any breath control necessary. Breathe normally, bringing full attention on the three phases of each step.

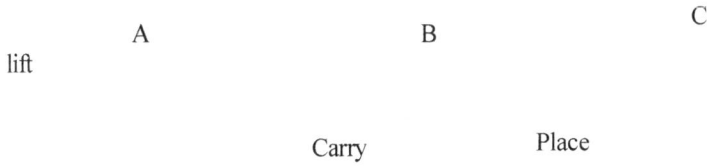

A   B   C
lift   Carry   Place

Each step has, first the lift (Fig A), second carry (Fig B) and third place on the ground again (Fig C). Start by lifting only your heel as the first impulse, toes still touch the ground, therefore lift means impulse of readiness. Do not lift the entire leg but be in a state of readiness by lifting only the heel (Fig A). The same foot is now carried forward, normally, not too high, nor too low (Fig B).

The second phase of carrying the foot forward now glides into the third phase. Place the foot firmly on the ground. Toes should first touch the ground and then the entire foot is firmly placed on the ground (Fig C) only to continue with the other foot, the same pattern of three phases - lift, carry and place.

Each step is magnified in time, so that each part of a step is brought into focus. This way one walks in continuum, in an awakened state, fully conscious of one's self, in togetherness with the environment. When you are at the end of your walk (at the other end of the room) continue the same backwards, without losing the rhythm which you have created – lift, carry and place.

Threefold walking (forwards and backwards) induces unity and harmonises your senses with each step. Gradually the thoughts will get focused, along with the entire organism in a state of totality. Do not limit yourself to any set time. End the exercise, whenever you feel like it. I have done this exercise on a number of occasions lasting from ten minutes to over an hour. It is a walk meditation, which creates calmness and a sense of inner space.

Do this exercise slowly and consciously to strengthen yourself and purify against mal (bad) aria (air). End it with IAO. This threefold walking exercise could also be used for Dengue, along with the IAO.

One more exercise, which works therapeutically for the symptoms of both Malaria and Dengue, is the resistance building movement called AA-Veneration.

Veneration is a state of mind, which enhances one's inner surrender to the essence behind the veil of existence. This inner surrender is not passive but asserts the smaller self-striving for the higher self, which connects all existence. AA is the open angled movement, which reaches out in wonder, in order to receive the beauty of creation, in deep veneration.

This resistance building exercise can be done best of all in the evening before one retires to bed, so that the forces of veneration can work in sleep and strengthen the immune system.

Stand normally with relaxed knees. Feel your feet grounded like roots of the tree. Now raise your arms upwards in an open gesture, feel or try to induce in yourself a feeling for a higher Being, for example, your Guardian Angel or any other Being you venerate (Fig 15).

15

With a small jerk of the shoulders allow your arms to bring downwards the lightfilled blessing of the Higher Being. Try to feel the stream of warmth, permeating all the way down to your feet. Stand quietly and feel this downward stream permeating you and repeat the exercise once again. Do not wait too long but repeat it at least six to nine times.

This exercise done every evening strengthens the resistance of your organism inducing healthy sleep.

Diarrhoea, Bilharzia and Schistosomiasis are highly differentiated symptoms but they all have one thing in common and that is, they are all metabolic digestive disorders.

In order to overcome the weakness and susceptibility of the digestive system in general, it is necessary to bring a boundary of strength and structure to your system. Thus, one has to create formative forces of the organism, in order to counteract the outflow of bodily fluids and to stabilise the metabolic digestive system.

The six positions given were founded by a German doctor and initiate called Agrippa of Nettesheim, born in Cologne (1486-1535). Much later, Dr. Steiner introduced special sentences in German, which are translated into English for each position. These words, sentences, should be said inwardly so that gradually one will feel the words whilst performing the sequence one after the other.

Start by standing with full attention on yourself. Do not close your eyes, breathe normally throughout the exercise. Close your feet, feel the ground.

I think speech	I speak	I have spoken

Take the first position, inwardly thinking the sentence: I think the Word or I think Speech. Hold the position briefly and glide on to the second position by shifting the right leg a bit apart, with the words: I speak. At the same time the arms are raised at the throat level.

The third position shifts the left leg a bit further lowering the arms at the level of the solar plexus, with the words: I have spoken. The fourth position shifts now the right leg a bit apart raising the arms above the head at an angle. The words are, I seek myself in the Spirit. In the fifth position, bring the left leg a bit closer to the right, lowering the arms at the head level, the words are: I feel myself in me.

I seek myself in Spirit	I feel myself within me	I am on the way to the Spirit

The sixth is the last position where the right leg joins the left, standing with closed feet and with the upraised arms together in parallel lines, with the words: I am on my way to the Spirit, within me. The last position ends with the arms raised upwards.

After holding all these positions briefly, take a small break and once more repeat the whole sequence from start to finish. Repeat the whole procedure five to seven times in succession and finish whilst standing quietly with full consciousness, ruminating the whole exercise inwardly.

This exercise creates a healthy foundation, which works against the overflow of precious bodily fluids. It is an excellent preventive exercise, also to encounter and counteract undue pressure of everyday life, which often sets chaos in our metabolic digestive system.

I come towards the end of describing Eurythmy exercises but for you it is the beginning. You have gained a different perspective and a new approach. Some exercises may appear complicated to begin with, but with patience and persistence you can perform them and overcome diseases in a holistic manner. Making a sincere effort, in itself, is therapeutical.

BRIEF NOTE ON HOW TO GET OVER JET LAG

In Ayurvedic parlance, the human body is regulated by *Kafa* (phlegm), *Pita* (bile) and *Vata* (gas). Any imbalance in these *tridoshas* (three humours) leads to diseases. *Vata* regulates respiration, excretion, nerve impulses, body movements and reflexes. Traveling causes vitiation of *vata dosha* which leads to tiredness, giddiness, disturbed sleep, nausea, headaches, arrhythmias, etc. The reasons could be varied, the jet speed of 1000 kmph as against the average speed of the body of 5 to 7 kmph, the less oxygen at 30,000 feet and above, cabin pressure, stress of travel, inadequate rest, change in food, etc. To counter jetlag, Eurythmy has different set of exercises, which are beyond the purview of this book. However, some suggestions are given below to keep you healthy during travels.

3 or 4 days before departure, after an early dinner, take a teaspoonful of any good unadulterated and undiluted potable lubricant like melted butter or olive oil. This helps to smoothen out and lubricate the inner lining of the digestive system and prevents congestion as well as constipation. This helps to maintain 'digestive rhythm' if one continues the same method 3 or 4 days after the flight. Also 2 or 3 days before departure, together with the above, massage your body, especially the soles of your feet, morning and evening,

to activate blood circulation. Any good oil will do, but refrain from perfumed or chemical based oils. This helps against dehydration of the skin and the 'added covering' works as further protection.

Do not forget to lightly massage your temples as well as the head, especially the top of the head, as this helps against susceptibility. You may lightly massage your head, neck and temples even during flight for added comfort and sound sleep. Drink lots of water to prevent dehydration. Fluid intake is most essential to strengthen immunity and flush out toxins. Avoid alcoholic drinks. Food intake during flights should be limited. These simple flight preparations, along with the basic Eurythmy exercises, strengthen the immune system.

- Dr. Leo Rebello

Naked Man and his Naked Madness

ANNEXURES

* Eat *Kanji* and Get Well
* Colloidal Silver,
* Korean *Kim Chi* or German Sauerkraut
* Medicine Madness
* Dr. Leo Rebello's Revised Oath for Doctors

This happy family will be extinct if we allow the bird flu racketeers to run amuck. Birds of various plumage have been with us for centuries. Do not panic by bird flu scare.

.... Dr. Leo Rebello

EAT KANJI AND GET WELL

Kanji (Indian word for rice cooked in 4-6 times its volume in water, till it becomes gruel), the simplest food known and savoured by human beings for centuries. Congee in English, Jook or zuk in China and Korea, Chao Bo in Vietnam, Lugaw in Philippines, Okayu in Japan, Khao Tom gung in Thailand. Served piping hot or 'overnight' cold. Fresh or fermented. Savoury, sweet or sour. Eaten with almost anything - eggs, chicken or shrimp, mushrooms, bamboo shoots or almost any vegetable. And sometimes, even with milk or coconut! Flavoured and spiced with almost anything - sesame seeds, dates, ginger, chili paste, garlic, black pepper, cumin or by itself, laced with a spoonful of ghee and a dash of salt.

Eaten as breakfast, lunch, brunch or dinner. Especially good when you're sick or cold or hungry or all three. Congee also refers to the starchy water that is drained off after rice is cooked. But here it is referred to as that wondrous, marvelous broth or rice gruel, as global as the UN, from Sydney to New York and Bombay to Brussels - there are even several restaurants dedicated to it! So, when you are down and out with tropical diseases, or any debilitating illness, take kanji and recover early.

Perhaps, one of the reasons for rice's hallowed, all pervading presence in our lives is because of its very high nutritional value. In Ayurveda, there are two grains in the list of earth's first foods - rice and barley. And so it is considered the perfect healing food. Brown rice, or rice with the bran and germ layers intact, for example, is one of the healthiest foods you can eat. It is low in fat, sodium and cholesterol. Being a slow digesting complex-carbohydrate, it is healthy and perfect diet to prevent and manage hypertension and obesity.

If you notice, predominantly rice eating societies both in India and the Far East have had fewer fat people, even though rice is eaten at every meal. And the misconception of rice being 'fattening' is because we eat it wrong and make it (and other nutritive foods like potato and ghee) the scapegoat for our sedentary, couch potato life styles. Brown rice is also high in Vitamin B complex and many vital minerals like selenium, magnesium and manganese.

Parboiled rice, India's contribution to world health, is one of the best kinds of rice for kanji. Milling and processing which makes rice 'white' does knock off 50 to 60 percent of many nutrients. But, one cup of white rice still gives 88 percent of the selenium in one egg, 80 percent B-complex vitamin (important in pregnancy and prevention of pregnancy defects) contained in one papaya and as much manganese as half a cup of spinach. In Ayurveda, white basmati rice is considered "easy to digest, cooling the digestive fires and held in high regard as a cleansing and healing food for all body types." Hence, many recipes in the Ayurvedic healing diet are based on basmati rice.

So, when rice is cooked to become rice gruel, all its nutritional benefits become available in a much more easy-to-assimilate and 98% digestible form. No wonder then that congee is considered everything from comfort food for the sick to nourishment for nursing mothers to a baby's first solid by Ayurveda, Siddha and Chinese and Tibetan medicine.

In Ayurveda, healing diets are considered absolutely vital during and after *panchakarma* treatments because of the need to cosset and mollify the body, mind and spirit of the patient. Of the 64 food preparations listed in the *shamana* or strengthening treatments, congee is one of them. It is prescribed during digestive ailments. For example, a version made with ginger and pomegranate juice is recommended in diarrhea and dysentery.

In Chinese medicine as in Ayurveda, wherein food is as much medicine as nutrition, congee occupies high place of importance. Combined with different foods it is used to treat a whole host of ailments: high cholesterol, insomnia, fever, to induce sleep and generally bolster weak constitutions. Congee with asparagus, for example, is believed to be a diuretic, while spinach congee is used as a sedative. In Basic Questions of Internal Medicine, also known as the Niejing, the basis of Chinese food therapy, written by Huang Di or the Yellow Emperor (27th century B.C.), he describes congee as "the most nourishing food on earth", because it is considered very nutritive and soothing for the digestive system and many problems related to it. That's why some Chinese claim it has the ability to bring back a person from the brink of death!

Edited version of Ratna Rajaiah's article published
in "Sunday" July 28, 2005.

COLLOIDAL SILVER

Edited version of article published by Health Freedom Resources, Inc.

Colloidal Silver is a near perfect antibiotic. Just about every known germ, bacteria, virus or fungus will die within six minutes of contact with c-silver. In addition, there are no known side effects. Silver can be used internally or externally.

For burns or sores that may be infected, use a wet bandage dipped in c-silver on the wound. On warts you can apply c-silver. Women suffering with a vaginal yeast infection can use 1 tablespoon of colloidal silver mixed in 8 oz. of water as a douche for almost immediate results.

For infectious diseases, c-silver can be taken internally either straight or mixed with liquid of choice. If you are dealing with an existing infectious condition, you may want to take 1 tablespoon of c-silver three times a day. As the condition improves you can reduce dosage to two tablespoons a day and then reduce to once a day. For general protection from colds, flu etc., a daily dose of one tablespoon is recommended.

"We have been using c-silver for about three years for various ailments. This weekend my son got very sick with a fever and sore throat and cough. I gave him 3 to 4 oz of c-silver water thrice a day, and in two days he was back to work with all the regular energy and no sickness. We also have pet animals and we give them c-silver water too. When our cow got sick recently we gave it c-silver instead of antibiotic and saw an amazingly fast recovery in just a day. That way we can still drink the milk. (You can't drink the milk of a cow on antibiotics)". D.E.

Colloidal silver was in common use until 1938 when the medical profession turned its attention to pharmaceutical drugs. An electro-colloidal process, which is known to be the best method, is most widely used now. The American Food and Drug Administration classifies c-silver as a pre-1938 drug. An antibiotic kills perhaps a half-dozen different disease organisms, but silver kills some 650. Resistant strains fail to develop. Moreover, silver is virtually non-toxic.

How it works
The presence of c-silver near a virus, fungus, bacterium or any other single celled pathogen disables its oxygen metabolism enzyme, its chemical lung, so to speak. Within a few minutes, the pathogen suffocates and dies, and is cleared out of the body by the immune, lymphatic and elimination systems. Unlike pharmaceutical antibiotics, which destroy beneficial enzymes, c-silver leaves these tissue-cell enzymes intact, as they are radically different from the enzymes of primitive single-celled life. Thus, c-silver is absolutely safe for humans, animals, plants and all multi-celled living matter

Ingesting C-Silver
Taken orally, the colloidal silver is absorbed from the mouth into the bloodstream, then transported quickly to the body cells. Swishing the solution under the tongue briefly before swallowing may result in faster absorption.

In cases of minor burns, an accumulation of c-silver may hasten healing, reducing the possibility of infection and scar tissue. (A fine spray mist or compress soaked in c-silver can also be very helpful.)

Chronic or serious conditions
One teaspoon of 10 ppm. c-silver equals about 50 micrograms (mcg.) of silver. One to three teaspoons per day (50 to 150 mcg.) is generally considered to be a nutritional amount and is reported to be safe to use for extended periods of time.

If your body is extremely ill or toxic, do not be in a hurry to clear up everything at once. If pathogens are killed off too quickly, the body's five eliminatory channels (liver, kidneys, skin, lungs and bowel) may be temporarily overloaded, causing flu-like conditions, headache, extreme fatigue, dizziness, nausea or aching muscles. Reduce the dose of c-silver and increase your distilled water intake. Regular bowel movements are a must in order to relieve the discomforts of detoxification. Resolve to reduce sugar and saturated fats from the diet, and exercise more. Given the opportunity, the body's natural ability to heal would amaze you.

Topical uses

Some have used c-silver in a nasal spray to reach the sinuses and nasal passages. Spray bottles have been used for topical use on kitchen and bathroom surfaces, skin, soar throat, eyes, burns, etc. C-silver is painless on cuts, abrasions, in open wound, in the nostrils for a stuffy nose, and even in a baby's eyes because, unlike some antiseptics, it does not destroy tissue cells. It's excellent as an underarm deodorant, since most underarm odor is caused by bacteria breaking down substances released by the sweat glands

Common uses of C-Silver

Colloidal silver can be applied directly to burns, cuts, scrapes, and open sores, or on a bandage for warts. It can be applied on eczema, itches, acne, sunburns or bug bites. To purify water, add one tablespoon per gallon, shake well and wait six minutes. Mixed this way it's tasteless. It is not an allopathic poison.

C-Silver Quality

Many brands of colloidal silver are inferior. The highest grade is produced by the electro-colloidal / non-chemical method where the silver particles and water have been collided, i.e., dispersed within and bound to each other by an electric current. The super-fine silver particles are suspended indefinitely in demineralised water. Ideally, c-silver is clear to a very slight golden yellow. Darker colors indicate larger silver particles that tend to collect at the bottom of the container and are not true colloids. If a product contains a stabilizer or lists trace elements other than silver, or if it needs to be shaken, it is inferior. If a product requires refrigeration, some other ingredient is present that could spoil. Some brands with high concentrations of silver may actually not be completely safe. The safe range of 5 to 15 parts per million (ppm.).

KOREAN KIM CHI
(German Sauerkraut)
by Dr. Leo Rebello

Prof. Timothy Watson, a Canadian based in Korea, for over a decade, wrote to me on July 24, 2005, that a report suggests that *Korean Kimchi* may have immunized Koreans against SARS since there were no cases of SARS reported in Korea. "It is the most powerful natural medicine", he says, "for bolstering and strengthening the immune system", and adds, "I can attest to this since I have not had any symptoms of bronchitis or serious colds since coming to Korea. My nail and hair growth is also substantially improved".

Kim chi is pickled or fermented cabbage. There are many different ways of making *kim chi,* and you can experiment as much as you want. A word to beginners: No matter whether Koreans are impressed with what you make even the most disappointing attempt at *kim chi* will taste great fried with noodles or rice.

You will need: * 2 Chinese cabbages. * 5-10 spring onions. * Sea salt or other non-iodized salt, at least 100 g. * 4 heaped tablespoons (about 20 g) Korean chili powder. * 2-3 cloves garlic, crushed. * 2 tablespoonfuls sugar, any kind. * 1 Tablespoonful kim chi sauce. * Small piece of ginger (5 g), crushed, or teaspoonful powdered ginger. * Half an onion (optional)

Rinse the cabbages, then quarter them lengthwise, discard the stems, and then chop the cabbages laterally, which should leave you with the largest pieces measuring perhaps 5 cm on a side.

Now that we have lots of little bits of cabbage, it's time to salt them. Place the cabbage in a clean plastic bag or equivalent (with no holes) and sprinkle salt over each layer. The best kind of salt is sea salt, although non-iodized table salt will do. This will create a brine solution with the cabbage juice. To ensure the cabbage is properly salted, sprinkle salt onto your wet hands, then rub it into the cabbage pieces. Press the leaves in your hand to squeeze as much water out of them as possible. Once finished, tie up the bag and set it aside for 5-6 hours. Check it after three hours to ensure that everything is all right, stirring the mixture if necessary.

Take the cabbage out of the salt solution and rinse it. It should be a lot softer than it was. Remove surplus water. Place cabbage in a sealable plastic box. Add the spring onions, chopped into small pieces. Crush the garlic and ginger in a press and mix in. You may also add half an onion, finely diced, if you wish.

Add red chili powder. Mash the chili powder into the leaves as you did in much the same way with the salt. If the color doesn't seem dark enough, add more chili powder. It's a good idea to wear gloves while doing this. Add two tablespoonfuls of sugar. You may also add *kim chi* sauce. Put the containers aside for three days. No snacking.

Finally the *kim chi* is ready. It should be soft in consistency, but not too mushy, with a little crunchiness left in the larger pieces. You can eat it as is, or mixed with other food. You can make *kim chi* from many other vegetables. You can add all sorts of things to the mix. The most common additional ingredients include 50-100g of finely shredded salted fish, scallops, or oysters.

Kim chi is called *Sauerkraut* in Germany, and according to some scientists it could be a secret weapon against SARS, Bird Flu virus. Their findings follow a study in which *kimchi* was fed to 13 chickens infected with bird flu. One week later, 11 of the birds showed signs of recovery from the virus.

Prof Kang Sa-ouk and his team of researchers from the Seoul National University claim that lactobacillus, the lactic acid bacteria created during the fermenting process, is the active ingredient that could combat bird flu and other type of flu viruses.

Health experts have already agreed that there may be some truth to kimchi's curative properties, prompting an increase in the consumption of the dish in South Korea. Whether or not sauerkraut does cure bird flu, the dish is said to have a number of other health benefits, among them cancer-fighting and detoxifying properties.

It is also a rich source of vitamins. One serving, which contains only 32 calories and has four grams of fibre, provides 102 per cent of the recommended daily intake of vitamin K, 12 per cent of iron and 35 per cent of vitamin C.

Prof Richard Mithen, from the Institute of Food Research, in Norwich, said: "Eating kimchi or sauerkraut may be good for your health and help fight off infections". Circulated on various d-lists in August 2005

A NOTE ON BIRD FLU
By Dr. Leo Rebello

Like SARS, Avian Flu is a false alarm. Don't panic, birds have been with us for centuries. Do NOT vaccinate them. Do NOT kill them in panic, for like the dead rat creates plague, millions of dead birds will create pandemic. Relax and do NOT fall a prey to this misleading propaganda. Above all, do NOT take Avian Flu shot, especially nasal spray. Because, then you will go on sneezing and spread the Avian Flu implanted in the shots by furious sneezing.

FOR FLU MY HOLISTIC TREATMENT IS: **(a)** Drink lots of citric fruit juices and clear soups. **(b)** No solid food for 3 days. *Kanji* may be taken, if absolutely necessary. **(c)** Warm Neem water bath will give refreshing feeling, especially when there are chills. **(d)** Lots of bed rest with windows open / no direct fan. **(e)** Morning sun bathing. **(f)** There are many homoeopathic medicines. I am giving only the main ones here. Head remedy: *Arsenic Alb* 30 - 4 hourly. Intercurrent remedy: *Influenzinum* 30 or 200 / 4 pills, 4 hourly - not more than 3 doses. For rapid prostration: *Kali Phos* 30 4 pills, 4 hourly. Stop once the patient feels better. *Pyrogenium* 200 / 4 pills, 3 hourly if severe back and thigh pains, extreme chilliness, rapid pulse. **(g)** The biochemic medicines are: *Ferrum phos*, *Kali mur* and *Natrum sulph* in 6 or 12 x potency 2 pills of each, 3 hourly. **(h)** Ginger, cinnamon teas with honey and a dash of sour lime are good. Even mint tea will soothe. **(i)** Fresh buttermilk, not refrigerated. Do NOT add sugar or salt. Similarly, one may take fresh coconut water.

MEDICINE MADNESS
By Dr. Leo Rebello

While in school, a mother dog had mildly scratched me (not bitten). This could have been treated with simple iodine or antiseptic wash. But the municipal hospital doctor, without asking me mandatory questions like whether the dog was rabid, whether it attacked without provocation, whether saliva dribbled from its mouth, etc. or without even examining me, jabbed me with two anti-tetanus and 14 mega painful injections on the abdomen, for 14 consecutive days. The treatment was much worse than the "dog bite". It is then I decided that I will become a better doctor and pursued Holistic Healing modalities.

If the diabetics have to live with insulin for lifetime, if asthmatics have to sleep with a pump, if high BP patients have to take anti-hypertensives for life, and others have to take anti-cholesterol, thyroid medicine, antacides for life; if cancer patients are made to suffer from chemotherapy (treatment worse than the disease); if the allopathic doctors have to depend on half a dozen dubious tests to determine whether it is malaria, typhoid, influenza or rheumatic fever before determining what fever it is; if by listening to medical representatives they prescribe inadequately tested and deleterious drugs, and if besides antibiotics, steroids and glucose saline they have nothing to offer, obviously it means that Allopathy is a bogus science.

This true story will shock you out of your wits. Circa 1981, at Bombay's biggest morgue in Government run JJ Hospital with bloated bodies stinking to high heaven, bandicoots and crows nibbling at the corpses, cockroaches and lizards, huge cobwebs, flies swarming, I saw one doctor working on a corpse with one hand and eating *batata wada* (big mack) with another!!! Eeek... I questioned him for the said act. He said he was hungry, tired and had to complete the assigned quota of bodies. In that case, I told him, you might as well eat in a toilet while attending to nature's call. He got the message. I also asked him what happened to his germs theory and antiseptic techniques, on which the whole edifice of modern medicine is based. He had no answer.

Later, I studied the racket called drug testing and found how FDA is the most corrupt organisation; how vaccines laced with themeserol/mercury created not only the diseases which they claim to prevent, but more lethal ones like Cancers, AIDS, Autism, Blindness, etc. Finally, the racket called HIV = AIDS and the free sale of ARTs and how WHO has become a 'WHOre' of the pharma mafia, CODEX manipulations, etc. Because of my fearless talk, they stopped inviting me to their conferences.

Earlier it was a lone battle. Now with the onset of the Internet, I am happy to say that awareness is growing and people are realising that modern medicine is the worst con. Today, there are many groups working against medical quackery. But I am the original quackbuster having started in early eighties. Like there are people who still think that to protect our borders we need huge armies and lethal arms, there are also 'brain damaged' (pun intended) people who run to ultra-modern hospitals and suffer in the process instead of introducing simple life-style changes.

In 1985, I wrote in an Editorial titled Health Care is Self-Care: "The present health system is top-heavy, over-centralised, heavily curative in its approach, urban and elite-oriented, costly and dependency creating. Unless it is community-based, people-oriented, economic, decentralised, democratic and participatory, we are afraid, the aim of the WHO to make available Health for All by 2000 AD will remain only on paper".

We are now in 2005, and instead of Health for All, it is Death for All with population control programmes like AIDS, Codex issuing a fiat that even vitamins, micro-nutrients will need doctor's prescription; compulsory and multiple vaccinations; children being prescribed in schools with downers for hyper-activity; airlines spraying chemicals (inside) to kill tiny insects and outside (chemtrails) to change the weather and destroy crops; difficult people (read those who can question) being asked to go in for psychological testing under the National Security Act; parents being prosecuted for shaken baby syndrome to cover the deaths due to vaccinations; parents not giving ARTs for AIDS facing jail term, America has become one massive concentration camp. Unfortunately British PM is dancing foxtrot with Uncle Sam.

With that hydraheaded monster called WTO spreading its tentacles, and neo-cons wanting to establish One World Order, the pharma-mafia, the petro-chemical mafia, the arms mafia, the World Bank mafia, gold syndicate, the drugs syndicate and other mafias are playing havoc with humanity.

Circulated worldwide through NGO-ICT (Japan), Zeus (London), Zest (Bombay) and published in Mangalore Today, July 2005 and in the book Free, Fair and Fearless, in December 2005.

REVISED OATH FOR DOCTORS
Ó Written and Administered by Dr. Leo Rebello, since 2003

This more comprehensive Oath was drawn by Dr. Leo Rebello in 2003, since Hippocrates Oath is now partly outdated being centuries old. This revised Oath has been widely circulated, accepted and appreciated.

1st July is celebrated as Doctors' Day all over the world. The day usually passes without a whimper. Many doctors have forgotten their Hippocratic oath or humanism. Therefore, I would like to administer the following oath to the doctors to serve as a reminder as to how important is their profession. Doctors to please repeat after me.

I, ——————, do hereby swear on this solemn day that :-
* I shall **not** prescribe unnecessary medicines and tests to my patients;
* I shall **not** give false counseling;
* I shall **not** overcharge and accept cuts and gifts;
* I shall **not** rape tiny tots with mercury laced innoculations or vaccinations, for they pollute the blood stream leading to serious diseases like AIDS, Cancers, Autism, etc;
* I shall **not** prescribe lethal drugs, like anti-retrovirals, chemotherapy, or give ECT to my patients;
* I shall **not** indulge in human organ thefts to the detriment of my patients;
* I shall **not** be afraid of any authority and fabricate medical records or give false evidence;
* I shall **not** exploit students studying under me;
* I shall **not** manipulate findings or results to win grants.

I, —————————, further solemnly affirm that:-

* If I cannot treat a disease, I shall **not** say that AIDS, cancers, diabetes has no cure. But will tell the patient to try other systems of medicine.

* I shall treat health practitioners of other systems with respect and **not** tell deliberate lies to prove my importance.

* I shall study Holistic healing modalities to increase my knowledge and wisdom.

* I shall **not** even by mistake say that "HIV=AIDS=Death" or cancers cannot be treated.

* I shall **not** frighten my patients with unnecessary comments, opinions or advice.

* I still remember what Hippocrates said, namely, "Let diet be your medicine" and shall accordingly prescribe fresh fruits, vegetables and good diet to my patients, rather than tonics, syrups, synthetic multi-vitamins, especially to children.

* I shall **not** perform surgery, unless it is absolutely must and will **not** indulge in rackets like amniocentesis, caesarian section, silicon implant or liposuction.

* I shall work to ban the useless and cruel animal experiments in the name of medicine.

* I shall participate in periodic workshops, seminars, conferences at my expense or on scholarship (no pharma funding) to educate myself and speak from my conscience if I am called upon to speak or preside.

* Finally, I shall not consume alcohol, smoke tobacco, or take other narcotic and psychtropic substances. As far as possible, I shall also not take animal proteins.

I realize and aver that a great responsibility of people's well-being is upon my shoulders and I shall carry on my onerous task with utmost dedication.

This I swear in the name of God on this solemn Doctors' Day and I shall repeat this oath daily lest I forget that I am in a divine profession to heal the world.

THE LAST WORD

If you have read this book fully, you would have noticed that whether it is dengue, *kala-azar*, malaria, typhoid, yellow fever, asthma, anemia, cancers, epilepsy or intestinal helminthiasis, the cause is a diseased colon, choked with faecal material, which is the root cause of all diseases.

We create the perfect living environment for parasites when the bowel becomes ineffective in the elimination of waste products. The build-up of faecal material on the walls of the colon is attributed to constipation and the amounts of junk food, chemicals, bad fats and sweets we consume. We poison ourselves from our own toxic waste.

Allopathy talks of incubation period for all diseases from 1 day to 1 year and more. That means, whatever goes into your body - including metals, gases – does not damage till it crosses the threshold. In other words, as long as your immunity is strong - and your immunity is based on your intestinal health, you are fine. **So, the simple message is: keep the colon clean and you will not have any problem.**

Drugs are not the answer to disease-strains. A pure blood-stream is the answer. Drugs cannot cure diseases; drugs multiply them. Allopathy has created about 30,000 diseases due to over use of drugs.

The basic difference here is between the holistic concepts of health care versus orthodox medicine's drug-oriented approach to disease care. The conflict is real: proper use of medications, diet, nutrition, and advice for the whole person as opposed to fancy bandaids that cover but don't cure disorders seen in isolated body parts.

Holistic healers view the body as a harmony of interacting processes, quite unlike conventional specialists who after medical school graduation take a body part – skin, bones, brain, heart, liver – or class of persons – babies, elderly, women – and go berserk with Louis Pasteur's plagiarized premise on which the entire rotten edifice of modern medicine is built. Holistic healing is more person-oriented than disease-oriented and consequently highly effective. Treatment programs arise from the idea that health care should take full consideration of human needs and be humane in attitude, ethics, and behaviour.

More than that, the holistic practitioner does not consider himself finished with his patient after providing 'technical services'. He is a counsellor who brings in other aspects of the individual's life, such as, his family and his community. They are a part of the larger whole, and each needs to be seen as interacting on that basis. The doctor helps to stimulate healthy interactions. In holistic healing, there is no 'active doctor – passive patient' role; the patient participates all the way as an equal-but-different partner.

Finally, the holistic healer actively informs his patients of issues they need to know related to their bodies, minds and the spirit. He recognises that his function is not merely that of a clinician and scientist but also that of a physician-teacher. At the very least, teaching might be by example – like *Irritable Bowel Syndrome* is largely due to the irritability of the mind.

Indeed, health education of patients and the public at large is the most important function of the holistic physician. This book proves the point by putting everything in proper perspective.

We choose our sickness when, through neglect or ignorance, we allow it to spread within us. Keep your body and mind clean and you will continue to be healthy without ills, pills and doctor's bills. Take Care.

Dr. Leo Rebello

THE HISTORY OF MEDICINE by Dr. Leo Rebello
2000 B.C. - Here, eat this root.
1000 A.D. - That root is heathen. Here, say this prayer.
1850 A.D. - That prayer is superstition. Here, drink this potion.
1940 A.D. - That potion is snake oil. Here, swallow this pill.
1985 A.D. - That pill is ineffective. Here, take this antibiotic.
2000 A.D. - That antibiotic doesn't work anymore. Here, eat this root.

BOOKS

AIDS and Alternative Medicine – Leo Rebello

Amrit Manthan (International Journal of Holistic Healing Arts) – Leo Rebello

Encyclopedia of A to Z Holistic Healing– by Leo Rebello (being compiled)

Free, Fair and Fearless -- by Leo Rebello

Nature Cure and Yoga Therapy – Leo Rebello

A Manual of Materia Medica Therapeutics and Pharmacy – A.L.Blackwood

Anthroposophic Medicine Today – Richard Leviton

Anthroposophical Spiritual Science - Rudolf Steiner

Comparative Materia Medica – E.A.Farrington

Concordant Materia Medica – Frans Vermeulen

Directory of Diseases and Cures in Homoeopathy – R.L.Gupta

Family Health Encyclopedia – A to Z Reference Guide by the British Medical Association

Fundamentals of Therapy - Rudolf Steiner and Ita Wegman

Homoeopathic Therapeutics – Samuel Lilienthal

Homoeopathic Repertory and Materia Medica – William Boericke

Indian Materia Medica – K.M.Nadkarni and A.K.Nadkarni

Man and Remedy – Special Issue of Weleda Newsletters for Physicians

Taber's Cyclopedic Medical Dictionary

Traditional Medicine and Health Care Coverage – WHO

SOFTWARE

Encarta Encyclopedia 2003. Microsoft Corporation.

Encyclopaedia Homoeopathica and Radar

WEBSITES

www.healthwisdom.org, www.emedicine.com, www.healthfree.com, www.itfnet.org/fruits.fm, www.tradewindsfruit.com/herbs, www.webhealthcentre.com, www.wikipedia.org

NOTE: We have not given **Glossary**. The medical words used in the book are clear in context. For the novice, 'Pocket Medical Dictionary' by Nancy Roper is good. Professionals may refer to Taber's Cyclopedic Medical Dictionary.